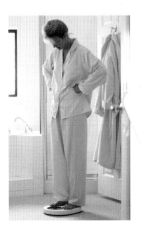

Natural
Menopause

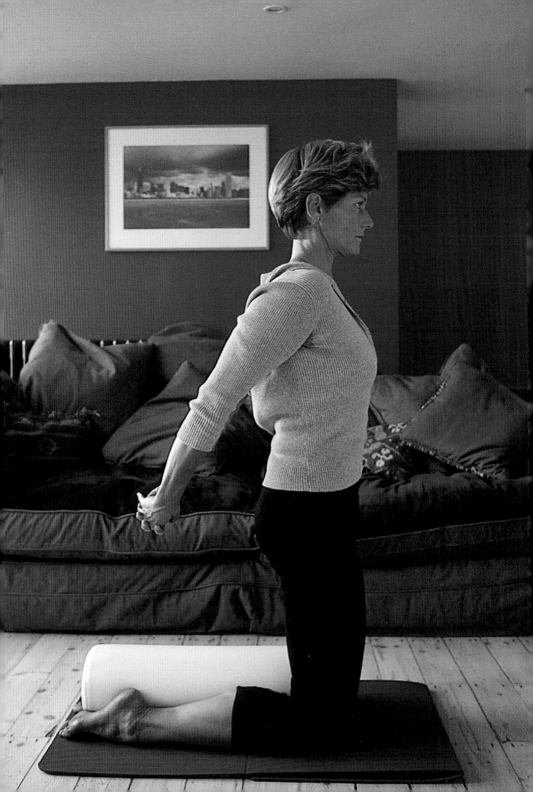

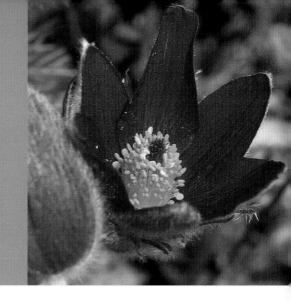

Natural
Menopause

Jan Clark

hamlyn

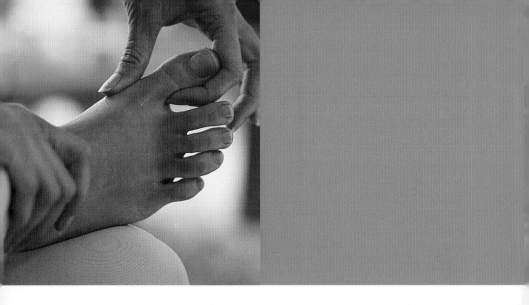

A Pyramid Paperback from Hamlyn

First published in Great Britain in 2004 by
Hamlyn, a division of Octopus Publishing Group Ltd,
2–4 Heron Quays, London E14 4JP

ISBN 0 600 61123 X

A CIP catalogue record for this book is available from the
British Library

Printed and bound in China

10 9 8 7 6 5 4 3 2 1

Safety note

While the advice and information in
this book are believed to be accurate
and true at the time of going to press,
neither the author nor publishers can
accept any legal responsibility or liability
for any errors or omissions that may
be made. The reader should always
consult a physician in all matters of
health and particularly in respect of
any symptoms which may require
diagnosis or medical attention.

Contents

Introduction

Menopause happens to every woman. Unlike other changes that affect a woman's body, such as pregnancy, menopause is something about which we have no choice. And that's why it's important to understand as much about it as possible.

Menopause is defined as 'the final cessation of menstruation', implying that it is like turning off the water tap one day. In reality, it's a much more gradual stop-start series of pauses in ovarian function which are part of the ageing process. Exceptions to this are women who undergo menopause suddenly, as a result of surgery, radiation therapy or chemotherapy.

Whether you experience menopause naturally or as the result of surgery, you will find it to be a uniquely individual experience. There are many myths and stereotypes surrounding menopause such as: women suffer from deep depressions and wild rages; they mourn their lost youth; or they lose the ability to have sex. In fact, the only universal statement that can be made about menopause is that menstruation stops. All the other particulars of the experience vary from woman to woman.

Derived from the Greek words *meno* (month) and *paussis* (pause), the term menopause was first used in 1872. At that time, Western medicine viewed menopause as a medical crisis that contained the potential for causing a variety of diseases, from diarrhoea to diabetes. In the middle of the 20th century, the medical profession switched from regarding menopause as the cause of disease and began to think of it as a disease itself. Now menopause is widely considered to be a natural event in a woman's life, and women living in developed countries can expect to live well into their 70s and 80s. This means that a full one-third of their lives will occur after their childbearing years are over.

In many non-Western cultures, menopause is viewed as a marker of increased social status. For instance, in Rajasthan, India, women who have gone through menopause may leave the women's quarters to talk and drink with men; among the Qemant people of Ethiopia, a woman who has achieved menopause is permitted to walk on sacred ground and participate in other rituals; while according to the traditional culture of the Cree in Canada, a woman who has passed through menopause may exercise shamanistic powers and play a direct role in religious ceremonies.

A positive change

The expectations that you have about the menopause will depend greatly on your own sense of worth and identity. Research has shown that the better a woman feels about herself and her life, the easier time she will have during menopause. In this book, I encourage you to value yourself and to have a positive attitude towards life. Many of the therapies I have included, such as meditation, yoga and massage, will help you to nurture yourself and enable you to achieve a deep sense of relaxation.

Menopause is a great time to cultivate new healthy habits – such as regular exercise – and give up destructive habits, such as smoking and not getting enough sleep. Taking the time to experiment with complementary and alternative remedies to help rebalance the body around its new hormonal state is not an issue of vanity, or of attracting potential lovers – it is an issue of physical and mental health.

This book is about choices to prevent and treat your menopausal symptoms naturally without resorting to hormone replacement therapy (HRT). The benefits and risks of HRT continue to be challenged in research findings, and there remains no consensus about the percentage of women who might benefit from it, the length of time for which it should be administered or the method of treatment. Given this uncertainty, it is hardly surprising that thousands of women are choosing to take control of their particular menopausal symptoms by using natural methods, rather than seeing them as a crisis requiring medical intervention.

Finally, menopause brings freedom from the emotional ups and downs that commonly accompany menstruation; it also brings the freedom to surrender to passionate love-making without the fear of pregnancy.

You have many years of productivity ahead of you. I hope you benefit from this book and can share it with someone close to you.

Menopause should be viewed as a positive life change.

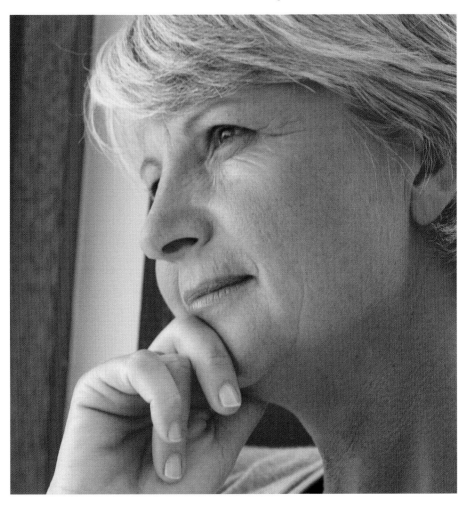

1

Natural Menopause

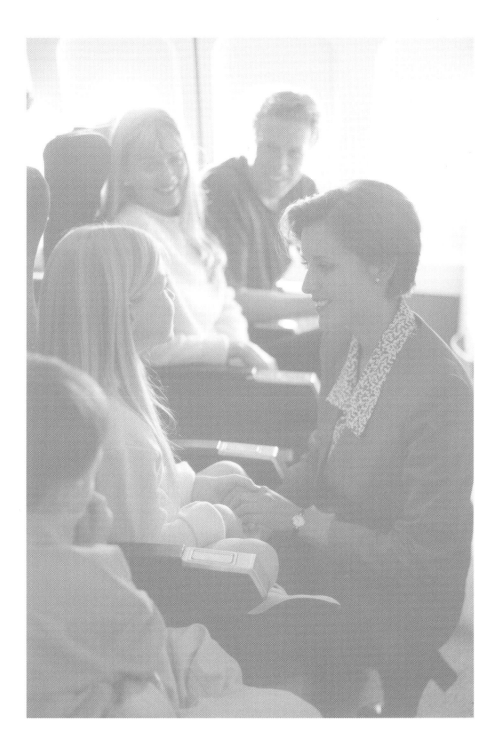

Hormones and your body

Perhaps you have picked up this book because you are suffering from menopausal symptoms, such as hot flushes and night sweats. They are interfering with your day-to-day life and preventing you from getting enough sleep at night. You feel it's time to take positive action and you want to know how you can alleviate your physical symptoms using natural remedies and complementary therapies.

Or perhaps you found yourself bursting into tears one day at work when your boss commented on your lack of concentration. It's true that your memory has not been as razor-sharp as usual. Now you want to find out how you can help yourself to control your moods and improve your memory and concentration.

Maybe you are shortly to have your ovaries surgically removed as part of a hysterectomy.

Taking time to pause and reflect on changes in your emotional and physical life can be very helpful.

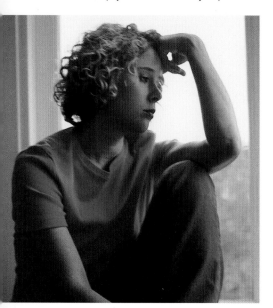

If you are premenopausal, this means you are likely to experience the onset of menopause within two years. Your doctor may have recommended that you take HRT to alleviate the symptoms. You haven't ruled this out yet, but you want to look into natural ways of managing your menopause.

THE ENDOCRINE SYSTEM

Hormonal highways develop through the endocrine system. This comprises a number of glands that produce hormones. The endocrine glands work as a team and include the following:

- **The pituitary** Located at the base of the brain, the pituitary is responsible for the secretion of two hormones essential to the reproductive system: follicle-stimulating hormone (FSH) and luteinizing hormone (LH). Its main activity is the control of the other endocrine glands.

- **The thyroid** Consisting of two lobes, one either side of the trachea (windpipe), the thyroid produces two hormones essential for normal metabolic processes and mental and physical development: T3 and thyroxine, or T4. T3 has a role in influencing mood and emotion, but its primary role is as an accelerator of metabolism in all organs of the body.

- **The parathyroids** Usually four in number and found on the back and side of each thyroid lobe, the parathyroids produce hormones that increase the amount of calcium circulating in the blood.

- **The adrenals** These consist of a flattened body above each kidney and are made up

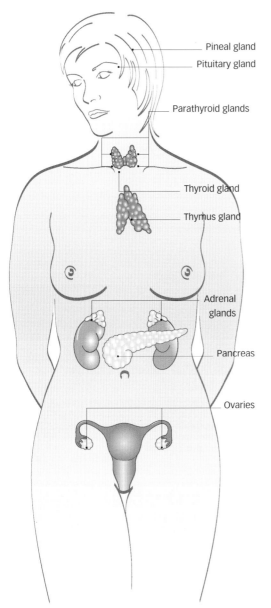

Pineal gland

Pituitary gland

Parathyroid glands

Thyroid gland

Thymus gland

Adrenal glands

Pancreas

Ovaries

of a cortex and a medulla. The adrenal cortex produces several hormones including cortisol (which is important in carbohydrate breakdown and in the normal response to stress) and the sex hormones (oestrogens and androgens). In men, androgens have an important role in stimulating the development of the sex organs and the principal source of these hormones is the testes. However, androgen hormones produced by the adrenals also have a vital role in women. After the menopause, some androgens, such as dehydroepiandrosterone (DHEA) and androstenedione, can be converted by the adrenals into oestrone, a weak oestrogen. This becomes the body's main source of oestrogen when the ovaries have stopped producing it. The adrenal medulla secretes adrenalin (epinephrine) involved in the 'flight or fight' response when in danger or under emotional or physical stress. A slow, rather irregular release of adrenalin goes on all the time, but a real boost to production is any situation fraught with fear or anger. When that happens, adrenalin increases the blood flow to the muscles by accelerating the heart rate and shutting off the less essential blood flow to skin and intestines.

• **The pancreas** This gland, which is located near the stomach, produces insulin, the hormone that regulates the level of sugar in the blood. Insulin works by making it easier for glucose to enter the cells, where it is used as fuel.

• **The ovaries** In addition to producing eggs, the ovaries produce the hormones oestrogen and progesterone (in response to FSH and LH from the pituitary gland) and testosterone.

WHAT ARE HORMONES?

The word hormone comes from the Greek word *horman*, meaning 'to stir up or arouse to activity', and this is exactly what hormones do. These chemical substances are made in minute quantities in glands, and circulate around the body via the bloodstream. Each one has a specific effect on its target organ or tissue, controlling, activating and directing structures and functions. Many hormones affect the urges, desires and feelings which are yours and nobody else's. Fluctuating hormone levels will vary throughout your life, influencing your moods, activities and sensitivities as they ebb and flow.

Hormones also:

- affect metabolic rate (how quickly/slowly you function)
- trigger growth (as at puberty – from about nine years old)
- balance blood sugar
- affect the body's water balance
- regulate respiration (your breathing)
- determine cell metabolism (the rate at which cells function)
- affect neural activity (your nervous system).

So you can see what a varied and complex part hormones play in your life and how much they matter. One hormone cannot be viewed in isolation but must be seen in its physiological context as a component in the whole balance of circulating hormones.

A QUESTION OF BALANCE

Some women live their whole lives with no hormonal problems whatsoever. Periods come and go with minimum disruption, pre-menstrual syndrome (PMS) is unknown, there is little or no trouble before and after pregnancy – even the contraceptive pill is swallowed without side-effects – and sterilization or hysterectomy produces no more than transitory difficulties.

But for other women, any interference with the hormonal system at any level causes chemical changes and alterations in body and mind rhythms, with resulting symptoms of hormonal distress.

Hormonal upset can arise from:

- the use of the birth control pill or other hormone-containing medicines
- hypothalamic or pituitary problems resulting from pregnancy, miscarriage or abortion
- surgery such as tubal ligation (sterilization) or hysterectomy
- anorexia or bulimia
- trauma (e.g. as a victim of violence)
- conditions such as ovarian cysts, polycystic ovaries, endometriosis or uterine fibroids.

Changes in hormone levels can also occur if the immune system breaks down as a result of chemical poisoning or viral infection, for hormonal problems and immune system dysfunction are often linked. For example, the main problem may be hormonal imbalance, but this is exacerbated by an impaired immune system function causing chronic tiredness. Or the basic problem may be centred on the immune system, causing damage to the ovaries and thus affecting hormonal status.

Stress and lifestyle will always play their part. For instance, female airline flight attendants frequently suffer menstrual instability because their biological 'time clocks' are disrupted as they fly through different time zones. Similarly, dancers, who need lean, muscular bodies, often experience amenorrhoea (an abnormal suppression or absence of menstruation). Traumatic experiences such as bereavement, divorce and violence all destabilize hormonal equilibrium, as can redundancy and moving home.

Frequent flying between different time zones can disrupt your biological 'time clock'.

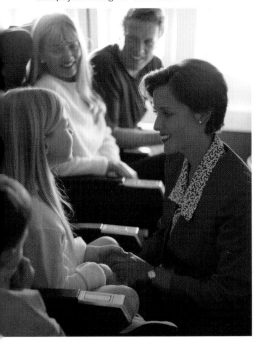

IT MAY BE IN YOUR GENES

Hormonal problems are often hereditary, so it is helpful to find out about your family's medical history. Often your mother's history and that of her female relatives can tell you a great deal about your own problems.

This can be especially useful if you are one of the 7–11 per cent of women who undergo a natural 'premature menopause' before the age of 40. Your hormone levels may appear normal, but you are experiencing typical physical and emotional symptoms of menopause, similar to those of family members.

OVARIAN CYSTS

An ovarian cyst is an abnormal, fluid-filled swelling that develops in the ovary. The most common type occurs when the egg-producing follicle of the ovary enlarges to produce a 'follicular cyst'. Cysts often produce no symptoms but some cause acute pain or irregular bleeding.

POLYCYSTIC OVARIES

This condition is thought to occur due to an imbalance between luteinizing hormone and follicle-stimulating hormone, produced by the pituitary gland. Multiple cysts develop in either one or both ovaries and ovulation ceases.

ENDOMETRIOSIS

This is a condition in which the cells that form the endometrium (lining of the uterus) develop outside their normal location, forming little clusters of tissue (called implants) outside the uterus.

FIBROIDS

These are lumps of fibrous and muscular tissue found growing on all levels of the uterus, although they have also been discovered in other areas within the pelvis. They are known to shrink naturally in women as they approach the menopause, but some researchers believe fibroids are sensitive to oestrogen and are more likely to grow when high levels of this hormone are present.

The ovarian hormones

Of especial importance to women are the three hormones produced by the ovaries: oestrogen, progesterone and testosterone.

OESTROGEN

Oestrogen is not really a single hormone: the word refers to a class of hormones that control female sexual development and promote the growth and function of female sex organs and secondary sexual characteristics. These oestrogens include the hormones oestradiol and oestrone, which are essential for the health of the reproductive organs, and oestriol, which is the predominant oestrogen hormone during pregnancy.

Your body began producing oestrogen when you were no more than a foetus, 15–20 weeks old, in your mother's womb. No doubt you

You can see how this baby's skin is beautifully soft and unblemished because of oestrogen.

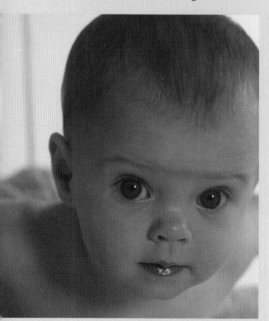

have marvelled at the exquisitely soft skin of a baby – this is due to oestrogen, which causes an extra layer of fat to develop and so makes the skin ultra soft.

At puberty, your level of oestrogen increased dramatically, albeit erratically: your breasts developed and the distribution of your body fat changed to produce the rounded contours of feminine hips and thighs – this is often described as 'puppy fat'. Maybe you can remember some of your emotions during puberty and adolescence – one day feeling elated and raring to go, the next apathetic and unhappy. These fluctuations are hardly surprising, given the bewildering and intricate changes that occur as your hormonal balance is established.

From this time your life became influenced by the cyclic monthly changes involved in menstruation as hormone levels rise and fall. For example, you may feel the stirrings of desire and the onset of sexual hunger in mid-cycle, at about the time your basal temperature readings indicate that you are at or near ovulation. This is the time at which both oestrogen and progesterone levels peak, indicating a readiness for pregnancy.

Oestrogen contributes to a healthy sex life, causing the vagina to moisten when aroused, and sensual areas to respond to stimulation.

As levels of oestrogen decline during the menopausal years, the vaginal tissues become thinner and dryer. Oestrogenic lubrication for sexual activity diminishes, and can result in vaginal penetration becoming uncomfortable or even painful.

PROGESTERONE

Progesterone is produced primarily by the ovaries, although smaller amounts are also produced by the adrenal glands and large amounts by the placenta during pregnancy. Its role is to maintain the healthy functioning of the female reproductive system.

At the time of ovulation, the ovaries dramatically increase their output of progesterone, stimulating a woman's sex drive and preparing the lining of the uterus for fertilization. Adequate levels of progesterone are essential to the survival of the fertilized egg and the foetus. They are also thought to be responsible for the sense of well-being that is experienced by some women during their pregnancies.

If you feel under par or even suffer pre-menstrual syndrome (PMS) at certain stages of your menstrual cycle, it is likely to be due to low levels of progesterone. It was the British gynaecologist Dr Katherina Dalton who pioneered the addition of progesterone for sufferers of PMS. She used to experience terrible migraines with her menstrual cycle and discovered these could be alleviated by progesterone injections. What led her to this discovery was the realization that her migraines completely disappeared during the final months of her pregnancy, which is when progesterone levels in the body soar. However, not all women in this situation respond in the way she did.

Apart from its reproductive function, progesterone is needed for the production of other hormones such as cortisol, which has an important role in the metabolism of carbohydrates, fats and proteins, and in the body's response to injury and infection.

The production of ovarian progesterone declines during the menopausal years as the reproductive process ends.

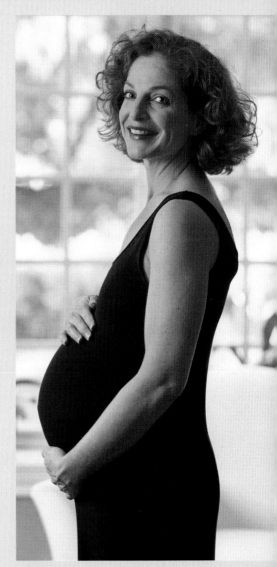

Hormonal balance contributes to the glow of healthy happiness seen in a pregnant woman.

TESTOSTERONE

As well as being a major hormone for men, testosterone is also of great importance for women. Not only are the levels of testosterone in women's blood higher than the levels of oestrogen, but their brains contain 20 times more testosterone than oestrogen.

Men have 10–20 times more free testosterone than women – one-half of a woman's testosterone is produced in the ovaries and the other half in the adrenal glands. The hormone helps to determine secondary sexual characteristics such as muscle mass and patterns of hair growth, and adequate levels are essential for sexual desire, activity and responsiveness in both men and women.

Nevertheless, while testosterone fuels the flames of desire, psychological factors determine the intensity and direction of the flame. The commonly held belief that hormones, in general, are the primary motivators of sexual activity in humans is a gross over-simplification: hormones do not cause behaviour, rather they raise the likelihood that a given behaviour will occur. Habit, circumstance, expectation and conditioning can all have a more profound effect on behaviour than hormones.

Testosterone levels reduce by about one-third in the average post-menopausal woman who still has her ovaries. If her ovaries are removed, the fall of testosterone is twice as great.

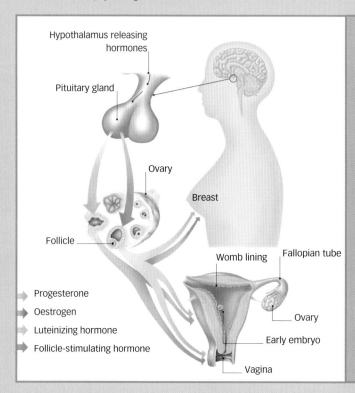

Hypothalamus releasing hormones

Pituitary gland

Ovary

Breast

Follicle

Progesterone

Oestrogen

Luteinizing hormone

Follicle-stimulating hormone

Womb lining

Fallopian tube

Ovary

Early embryo

Vagina

THE HORMONE LOOP

Throughout the month, a constant feedback loop creates a continuous adjustment and regulation of the hormone levels between the hypothalamus and pituitary, and the ovaries.

The change

The three hormones described on the preceding pages – oestrogen, progesterone and testosterone – constantly change from day to day in a predictable and orderly rhythm. They are key to the years during which a woman is at her reproductive prime. This is a process with a beginning, a peak, a decline and an end – and, interestingly, humans are the only mammals in the world to experience this, all other female mammals continue to reproduce until they die.

Central to a woman's reproductive life are her two ovaries. Estimates vary, but it is believed there are 6–7 million eggs present in a female foetus by the middle of its gestation. These begin to die off even before the child is born, but even so, the ovaries at birth contain somewhere between half-a-million and five million eggs. As the child develops the eggs continue to die off, so that by the time she reaches puberty there are between 200,000 and 300,000 eggs.

Each time a woman ovulates, not one or two, but between 20 and 1,000 eggs are used

During a woman's fertile years, one of her ovaries will ripen and release an egg once a month.

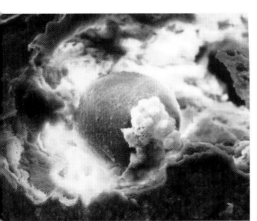

up. Only one or two eggs per cycle would have fully matured, and with increasing age the eggs become used up more rapidly. Between the ages of 38 and 44, about 50,000 eggs are lost.

Ovulation slows down during the peri-menopause: this is defined as the transition between the time you begin to experience menopausal symptoms (usually the mid- to late 40s) and the time when your periods actually stop (average age 51).

Many women find that they experience the menopause at the same age as their mothers.

HOW DO I KNOW IF I'M IN MY PERI-MENOPAUSE?

The signs that herald the arrival of the peri-menopause are varied. You might find yourself having two periods a month, and if you get a heavier flow, you may think you are always bleeding. Or you could go several months without bleeding. The actual flow may change, with lighter, more watery bleeding and less clotting due to reduced oestrogen levels. The hormone-related symptoms of the peri-menopause can be bothersome and include:

- night sweats, interrupted sleep or insomnia
- irritability and mood swings
- anxiety
- loss of concentration
- headaches (especially pre-menstrual migraines)
- vaginal dryness
- vaginal atrophy (thinning of the vaginal walls due to lack of oestrogen)
- less interest in sex
- urinary stress incontinence.

Many symptoms are interconnected. For instance, if you have such severe night sweats that you develop insomnia, your concentration will suffer and you will be irritable.

REVERSE PUBERTY

Any mood swings may well strike a chord with your early adolescence. The fluctuating hormonal levels, coupled with the daily traumas of adolescent life, lead to the wild mood swings that are so much a part of being a pubescent girl. In the peri-menopause, the exact reverse happens but with similar results: the ovaries are winding down instead of gearing up, but the duelling hormonal levels can bring on the same mood swings you probably experienced all those years ago.

IS IT HOT IN HERE TODAY?

The most commonly experienced peri-menopausal symptoms are hot flushes and night sweats. These occur in up to 25 per cent of peri-menopausal women and 50–85 per cent of menopausal women experience them. For most women, they happen over a period of one to two years, but in 20–25 per cent they continue for more than five years. A sudden hot flush can cause considerable surprise and embarrassment. One day you are busy in the office as usual, the next moment you suddenly feel a warm sensation rising up from your chest, spreading across your neck, up to your head and scalp... it's boiling hot in the room, beads of perspiration prickle your skin. After what seems an age, the heat is gone, you are wet with sweat and almost immediately you begin to feel chilled.

A typical hot flush lasts no more than three minutes, but it can range in duration from a few seconds to half-an-hour. It can be experienced in different ways. Some women have a specific focal point, such as the skin between the breasts, where the first tingles

The sudden onset of a hot flush can be very unsettling.

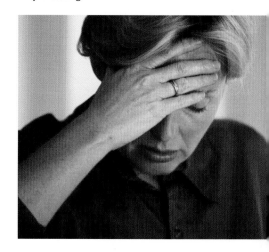

are felt, warning of an approaching hot flush. There may be no outward sign of redness or sweating – or you might sweat profusely and become as red as a beetroot. The degree of sensation varies from mild discomfort to such intense feelings that you have to fight the urge to pull off your clothing.

At night, the flushes are called night sweats, and you may wake up to find yourself drenched in sweat, and need to dry yourself and change your night clothes. Women often complain that night sweats are worse than daytime flushes because:

- it is not possible to pick up the warning signals of an approaching flush while asleep, and do anything to lessen its impact
- disturbed sleep results in tiredness, depression and irritability the next day.

Why do hot flushes happen?

The physiology of hot flushes is not yet fully understood, but they are due to chemicals being released into the bloodstream at this time of hormonal disruption. The blood vessels are sensitive to the chemicals and dilate, so blood rushes to the skin, making you hot and red. A medical dictionary defines hot flushes as 'vasomotor symptoms of the climacterium – sudden vasodilation with a sensation of heat, usually involving the face and neck, and upper part of the chest; sweats, often profuse, frequently follow the flush'.

Hot flushes are termed 'vasomotor' symptoms because the size of the blood vessels changes as part of the body's temperature-control system – blood vessels dilate (get larger) to allow more blood through so that you can cool down. They are linked to the breakdown of temperature control by the hypothalamus as oestrogen production declines. Hot flushes signal the completion of your life as a potential bearer of children for, at or near your menopause:

- your ovaries have used up all their eggs
- they therefore no longer respond to the secretion of FSH from the pituitary as they once did by producing oestrogen.

COMPLETING MENOPAUSE

A few women go through the peri-menopause overnight – periods will simply cease and these women have no associated symptoms. But most women experience some discomfort at this time and are aware of hormonal changes going on within their bodies which may or may not disrupt their lives. This is usually an erratic process: periods may come late or early, may be short or long, light or heavy – or vanish for months and then suddenly reappear. It can take between two and five years to complete and enormous changes take place in a woman's body as it acquires a new balance with lower levels of hormones.

The menopause is considered complete when periods have not occurred for one year.

Emotional distress

Everyone is aware of physical symptoms of the menopause, such as hot flushes and night sweats, but menopause can also be a time of great emotional upheaval. Mood swings, feelings of sadness, anxiety, stress and irritability are all common. You may also find your sense of identity changes as you come to the end of your reproductive years.

Some women find that the emotional symptoms of the menopause are compounded by stresses at work or at home, such as caring for elderly parents and teenage children. If you are accustomed to putting everyone else's needs – including those of your partner – first, you may find yourself drained of resources. The menopause is a time when your vulnerability needs to be acknowledged. Here are some suggestions about how to look after yourself:

- Visit your doctor and obtain advice about your menopausal symptoms.
- Arrange a family get-together. Let them know how you are feeling physically and emotionally. They will be much more understanding about your menopause if you share your distress with them, especially when they realize it will not last forever.
- Now is the time for domestic and any other family responsibilities, including caring for an elderly parent, to be shared out between you all.
- Set aside 3–4 hours in the week that are purely for you: you might choose the luxury of a pampering facial and/or a massage, swimming, yoga classes or a long lunch with friends.

THE END OF FERTILITY

If you have had all the children you wanted to – or if you chose not to have children – the fact that your childbearing years are coming to an end may not feel particularly significant. If, on the other hand, you wanted children (or a larger family than you have), the menopause may be a time when you find yourself grieving for the children you didn't have.

If part of your menopausal distress involves thinking about your childlessness, you can help to resolve this by writing about your thoughts and feelings in a letter to your unborn child. Tell your 'child' about yourself, your family, your hopes and dreams, and what you might have shared and enjoyed together. You may decide to write this letter all at once, or gradually over a few weeks. Once you have finished, put all the pages in a large envelope, perhaps with some family photos and drawings, and tuck it all away in a drawer. Creating something special out of your sadness will help you move towards resolving this emotional distress.

> " *I became aware of changes going on within me when I was 48. I still had two children, aged 23 and 25, living at home, as well as a teenage daughter. I would start weeping for no apparent reason, and didn't want to get out of bed most days. I was incredibly irritable with all the family, shouting and nagging them on the slightest pretext. My elderly widowed mother, then 82 and living a mile away, expected my undivided attention, especially as I was her only child, and I could not say 'no' to her demands.*
>
> **MARYANN (Cardiff)** "

MENOPAUSAL SYMPTOM CHART

Tick the box that most closely reflects how severely you are experiencing each of these symptoms. Each box you ticked has a score beside it.

Symptoms	Severe	Moderate	Mild	None
Hot flushes	12 ☐	8 ☐	4 ☐	0 ☐
Sweating attacks	12 ☐	8 ☐	4 ☐	0 ☐
Tension/irritability	3 ☐	2 ☐	1 ☐	0 ☐
Dryness of vagina/irritation	3 ☐	2 ☐	1 ☐	0 ☐
Loss of interest in sexual intimacy (ignore if not applicable)	3 ☐	2 ☐	1 ☐	0 ☐
Insomnia	3 ☐	2 ☐	1 ☐	0 ☐
Lack of energy	3 ☐	2 ☐	1 ☐	0 ☐
Hair/skin changes	3 ☐	2 ☐	1 ☐	0 ☐
Muscular and/or joint pains	3 ☐	2 ☐	1 ☐	0 ☐
Changes in memory/concentration	3 ☐	2 ☐	1 ☐	0 ☐

Once you have ticked a box for each symptom, add up your score.
A score of 30 or more strongly suggests that symptoms are associated with the menopause, although a low score will not exclude this.

Surgical removal of the ovaries

For some women, removal of the ovaries may be the only option if severe symptoms of pain, PMS or endometriosis persist and all other treatments have been tried or if the ovaries are diseased.

Endometriosis is a disease affecting many women in their reproductive years and it will recur while there is ovarian function. Although the ovaries themselves may be healthy, surgery involving hysterectomy and removal of the ovaries is the only permanent cure. Endometriosis is the only disease that is 'treated' by the surgical removal of tissue not directly affected by the disorder.

You are likely to be prescribed hormone replacement therapy following removal of the ovaries, but some doctors advise against HRT for the first six months. If all the endometrial implants are removed during the operation, then the chance of a recurrence of the disease is slim – however, if even the tiniest deposit remains, then HRT will assist its growth.

All too often, removal of ovaries is recommended for women aged 50+ who are having a hysterectomy, on the grounds that ovarian cancer may develop if they are retained. There is still considerable controversy about this issue, and if you are faced with this possibility, you need to weigh the risks of developing ovarian cancer against the benefits of continued ovarian function (that is, hormone production). The latest research in the USA, Denmark, Japan and Australia, as well as that undertaken by Cancer Research in the UK, indicates the following:

- Family risk factors include infertility, a well-documented history of ovarian cancer, late menopause and lack of child-bearing.
- Hysterectomy may reduce the risk of ovarian cancer by 36 per cent (although the Danish nationwide controlled follow-up study of ovarian cancer after hysterectomy (1997) suggests this protection might fade out with time).
- Women preserving at least one ovary have a significantly decreased risk of suffering from ovarian cancer for at least ten years after hysterectomy.
- Women who had heavy periods before hysterectomy tend to have a lower risk of ovarian cancer after surgery than women who had light or normal periods.

PREMATURE MENOPAUSE

Whether you are 20 or 50 years old, surgical removal of the ovaries is a very serious step to take. It leads to a premature menopause either straightaway or within two years of the operation, and you are likely to be prescribed HRT. This may result in months of trial and error until the correct dosage is found to supplement your own reduced oestrogen levels.

IMPORTANT

It is vitally important that you discuss all the issues and implications of HRT in detail with your doctor if your ovaries are to be surgically removed.

If you are still ovulating, then removing your ovaries will deprive you of significant hormonal support which is difficult to replace adequately. The most critical issue is loss of bone mass leading to osteoporosis, which surgical removal of ovaries is known to initiate (see page 32). In menopausal years, the ovaries continue to secrete hormones which will support your well-being and health.

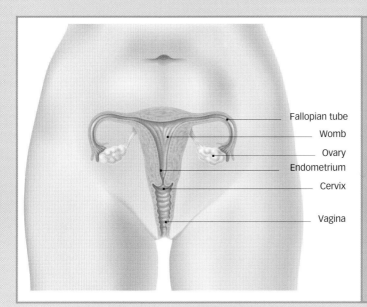

Fallopian tube
Womb
Ovary
Endometrium
Cervix
Vagina

THE REPRODUCTIVE SYSTEM

The main components of the reproductive system are the womb (uterus), fallopian tubes and ovaries. The outlet of the womb is the cervix, which projects downwards into the vagina.

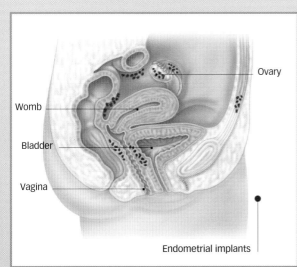

Ovary
Womb
Bladder
Vagina
Endometrial implants

ENDOMETRIOSIS

The diagram indicates some of the internal organs where deposits of endometriosis are commonly found.

2
Taking care of your body

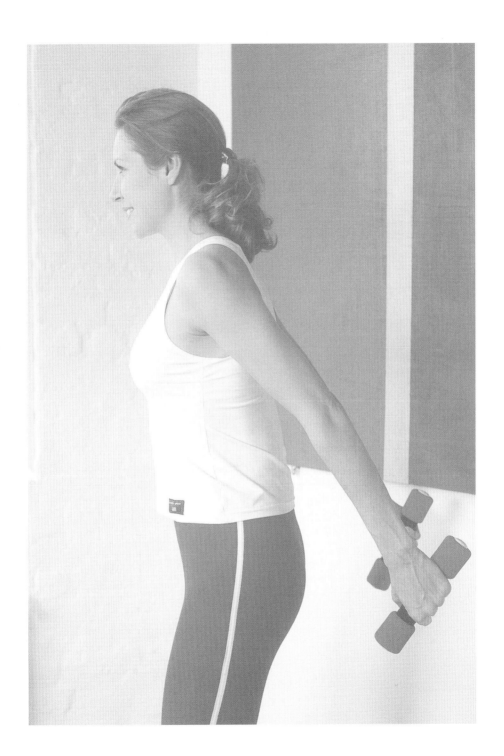

The missing hormone - natural progesterone

In the early 1900s, research into the mysteries of women's hormones first revealed the existence of oestrogen. Further investigations identified a second hormone which was necessary to maintain a successful pregnancy: this was named progesterone (pro-gestation).

In the 1970s, following years of research, Dr Ray Peat – a biochemist from Oregon – became convinced that progesterone was a very important hormone for osteoporotic post-menopausal women, as it could actually stimulate the formation of new bone. Furthermore, he claimed that progesterone could be made from yams, soy, and indeed 5,000 different plants.

It was found that one of the richest sources of progesterone for commercial use was a substance called diosgenin, found in the Mexican wild yam (*Dioscorea villosa*) – not to be confused with the average supermarket yam, which is really a sweet potato.

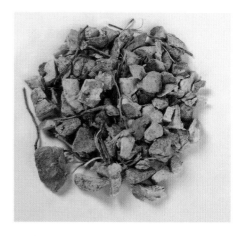

Mexican wild yam (*Dioscorea villosa*) contains a substance called diosgenin.

The discovery that diosgenin could be easily converted into a molecule that is identical to progesterone made by the body paved the way for progesterone creams (or gels) that could be smeared on any soft skin, such as a woman's tummy, inner thigh or breast. The commercial bandwagon swung into action – huge farms growing wild yams sprang up in Mexico.

The evidence for the efficacy of progesterone cream is mixed. In trials, women receiving progesterone transdermally have reported relief from menopausal symptoms such as hot flushes and breast tenderness. However, there is less evidence that progesterone can help osteoporosis by increasing bone density.

A NATURAL HORMONE?

Some of the assertions about yams and progesterone were refuted in *The Yam Scam* by American doctor John Lee. He argued that

TESTING TIMES

After three months of treatment for menopausal symptoms in a double-blind placebo-controlled study using a topical product containing wild yam, researchers at the Baker Medical Research Insitutute, Melbourne, Australia, found no statistical difference between placebo and active creams, even though 'mood swings' of women using the active cream actually improved in this trial. The ingredient responsible for this may well have been the geranium essential oil used in the cream.

> **"** *Four years ago menopausal symptoms such as mood swings, forgetfulness, lack of focus, vaginal dryness and discomfort were driving me crazy. My family medical history contraindicated HRT - Mum had high blood pressure and a stroke when she was 60, I had had a breast lump and a malignant melanoma on my wrist. I read about progesterone in a health magazine, and within days was using a progesterone cream – I think it is fantastic, it has regulated all the problems I had.*
>
> FIONA (Cambridge) **"**

the human body is unable to convert diosgenin in yam plants to progesterone. In addition, progesterone creams do not contain any wild yam at all – the main manufacturers use soya beans. Indeed, Dr Lee goes on to say that:

- progesterone itself is not found in wild yams
- it is synthesized from the plant material by a number of chemical steps, which means it is not 'natural' at all
- a chemical conversion process is necessary to synthesize progesterone from diosgenins, and this can only be done by a chemist in a laboratory
- as the progesterone did not dissolve well in alcohol, and any solvents tried were highly toxic, a method was patented for dissolving it in Vitamin E.

Despite evidence to the contrary, there are thousands of menopausal women who report that natural progesterone products have a beneficial effect on their symptoms.

AVAILABILITY OF PROGESTERONE

In the UK, progesterone cream is available only on prescription, although it can be purchased via websites or by mail order. In the USA and in most other countries, progesterone cream is available without prescription.

Progesterone-containing remedies come in three main forms: creams, granules and oils. The granules and oils have at least three times the concentration of progesterone found in the creams. They are taken by putting a few drops of the oil or several of the granules in the mouth and holding them under the tongue, usually for 5–8 minutes, until they have been absorbed by the lining of the mouth. Progesterone gets into the bloodstream straightaway when it is taken like this. Progesterone creams are effective for long-term use and maintenance.

ARE THERE ANY SIDE-EFFECTS?

Natural progesterone is not known to have any side-effects, except for altering the menstrual cycle temporarily in some women and bringing about feelings of euphoria.

Very occasionally, a post-menopausal woman will experience a small period for the first month or two, then this stops permanently. Should this happen, it is a sign that the progesterone is causing your body to eliminate excess stored oestrogen, which can trigger a shedding of the endometrium or 'breakthrough bleeding'. If any kind of breakthrough bleeding continues for more than three months, it is important to consult a doctor.

DID YOU KNOW?
At present the UK National Osteoporosis Society medical advisers do not consider there is enough valid scientific evidence to recommend the use of natural progesterone creams to prevent osteoporosis.

Sex and the menopause

You may have a happy and healthy sex life throughout your menopausal years. Alternatively, your sex drive may diminish or you may, through choice or circumstance, be outside of a sexual relationship.

USE IT OR LOSE IT

Regardless of whether you have sex with a partner, your vaginal health is important during and after the menopause. Most of the benefits of sexual stimulation, such as increased glandular and circulatory activity in the pelvic region, can be just as easily achieved through masturbation as they can through intercourse. Stimulation and orgasm – not the presence of a partner – are what keep your vagina healthy.

When ovarian function ceases, the loss of oestrogen can affect the appearance and sensitivity of your genitals. Like all menopausal symptoms, some women experience this to a greater degree than others. Some women are completely unaffected.

The first changes you may notice are in your outer genitals. Pubic hair thins and the labia lose fat tissue. Your vaginal lips become less full and less responsive to touch. Inside, the walls of the vagina thin and become more fragile as a result of decreased blood supply.

If your vagina is not stimulated through sexual play or masturbation, the diminished blood circulation to your genitals eventually affects your nerves and glands in this area. As the nerves lose function, there is less sensation during sex, and as the glands lose function, you produce less lubrication when you are aroused.

A downward spiral

If you notice a decline in the sensitivity of your genitals, you may well avoid intercourse, perhaps thinking 'why bother?' But abstinence accelerates the cycle of deterioration and your vagina will become smaller and less elastic, a condition known as vaginal atrophy. This means that any attempts at intercourse in the future will result, at best, in no feelings at all and, at worst, in pain. In extremely severe cases, the vagina can tear during intercourse. In addition, the acid/alkaline balance in the vagina alters from a fairly acid one to an alkaline environment, and the latter makes infections more likely. All these physical changes to your genitals can result in:

- diminished response to sexual stimulation
- reduction in reaction time of the clitoris
- difficulty in achieving orgasm
- increased susceptibility to infections: if you have an atrophied vagina you may be prone to vaginal inflammation, itching and discharge.

THINK SEXY!

Attitude is everything. Your mind has a powerful effect on sexuality, and your brain remains your chief sexual organ. If physiology were the sole component of sexuality, we would all crave exactly the same amount of sex, and lose interest at the same time and at the same rate. That simply does not happen.

Upward solutions

Start with an over-the-counter lubricant for your vagina, such as K-Y jelly. Although it will not reverse thinning of or damage to the vaginal walls, a lubricant will certainly make sex more comfortable.

Sexual play which includes cunnilingus (sexual stimulation of your genitals by your partner's lips and tongue) can be very arousing and helps to increase the blood supply and lubrication to your genitals.

If you've noticed a slowdown in sexual response time, try oral sex, mutual masturbation or a vibrator. During menopause you may require more direct stimulation of your clitoris in order to reach orgasm.

CONTRACEPTION DURING THE MENOPAUSE

Technically, menopause means a lack of menstruation for 12 months. Because this can only be determined retrospectively, using some form of contraception is advisable unless you have been sterilized, had a hysterectomy, or your male partner has had a vasectomy.

PREVENTING STDs

If you are having sex with a new partner, it is always sensible to use condoms to prevent the transmission of sexually transmitted diseases (STDs).

Hormonal contraception

The combined Pill (containing ethinyloestradiol and progestogen) was traditionally considered unsuitable for older women, and many women were advised to stop taking it at the age of 35. Now research has shown that, providing there are no contraindications, the combined Pill can be used by women up to the age of 50 with very low risk to health and even some benefits.

The mini-Pill (or progestogen-only Pill) has long been considered suitable for older women and is as effective as the combined Pill. Women often move from a combined to a progestogen-only Pill when they reach 35 and/or if they are smokers, obese, suffer from migraine or have raised blood pressure or a family history of heart disease.

Missed periods are very common on the mini-Pill and may worry you. You should tell your doctor if you start to bleed between periods – a change to another contraceptive method may be recommended.

Barrier methods

The cap or diaphragm is a rubber device which is squeezed into place to block the passage of sperm through the cervix at the top of the vagina. It should be used with a contraceptive jelly to seal the gap between the edge of the device and the vaginal wall. You should insert the cap or diaphragm before sexual intercourse, or before you go to bed, and remove it six hours after intercourse.

Your doctor will examine you to see which size cap or diaphragm you need, and show you how to insert it. After a trial period, you will have a check-up to make sure you are using it correctly. This is followed by yearly check-ups.

One advantage of the cap or diaphragm is that it holds back the flow of menstrual blood if you have intercourse during your period. This is useful at menopause when your periods may be unpredictable.

The sheath or condom is the most popular and easily available contraceptive method of all. It is like a second skin that is rolled over the erect penis before penetration and discarded after withdrawal.

DID YOU KNOW?

None of the natural methods of birth control, such as the calendar method, the temperature method or the cervical mucus method, are recommended for menopausal women. This is because ovulation occurs erratically at menopause, making it hard to tell when you are fertile.

The misbehaving bladder

During your menopausal years, you may find yourself going to the bathroom more often than when you were younger. Or you may find your body leaking small amounts of urine when you sneeze, cough, laugh or exercise. This problem, known as urinary incontinence, is quite common, although many people find it embarrassing to talk about.

Both men and women may experience reduced kidney function as they get older. The ureter (the tube that carries urine from the kidney to the urinary bladder) narrows and contracts. The possible results of this are:

- Urethritis (inflammation of the urethra)
- Repeated bladder infections
- Inflammation of the ureter
- Painful or difficult urination
- A triad of urinary problems: urgency, frequency and incontinence

As you get older, your bladder may also feel as though it needs emptying when it is only half full. As a result, you will need to urinate more frequently. Urinary incontinence has a variety of causes:

- The muscles of the pelvic floor and abdomen sometimes weaken with age, particularly in women who have had several children. This loss of muscle tone can lead to urine leakage when there is increased pressure on the bladder, for example, when laughing or coughing.
- Repeated bladder infections.
- Incontinence can occur in certain illnesses, such as Parkinson's disease, diabetes and bladder cancer.
- Women who have had a hysterectomy sometimes experience incontinence, both post-operatively (when it is usually transitory) and at menopause. This is either because their urinary structures have begun to drop down after bearing many children, or because the removal of the uterus has left the bladder and urethra without support. In rare cases, the urinary tissues may have been damaged during surgery – it is not unknown for the ureter to have been cut accidentally by the surgeon.

URGE INCONTINENCE

This means leaking urine when you feel the need to go to the toilet, perhaps as you are on your way to the bathroom. Urge incontinence is common around the menopause and 70 per cent of ageing women have it to some degree. Urge incontinence, which may also be associated with bedwetting at night, indicates lessened residual volume – this means that the volume of urine that the bladder can hold has decreased.

STRESS INCONTINENCE

This means leaking urine when coughing, sneezing or straining, and is often connected with uterine prolapse in women. The bladder is not able to hold as much urine as it previously could. Stress incontinence is not associated with bedwetting problems at night.

OVERFLOW INCONTINENCE

This is more common in men than women and is usually due to swelling of the prostate gland and incomplete emptying of the bladder. There is a sense of fullness or a 'need to go' but difficulty in actually urinating.

A 'misbehaving bladder' can be helped by a good urologist, but you may decide to try some of the following self-help measures first:

- You are more likely to have problems with incontinence if you are overweight. Extra abdominal fat puts too much stress on the bladder and urethra and causes them to sag down and leak. Losing weight will improve this situation.
- Watch what you eat. Some foods, such as citrus fruit and spicy foods, can irritate the bladder and worsen the problem of leakage.
- Cut back on your consumption of caffeine and alcohol.
- Strengthen your abdomen and pelvic muscles by doing Kegel exercises.
- Review any prescription drugs with your doctor. Some drugs, such as antihistamines and tranquillizers, can cause or aggravate bladder-control problems.

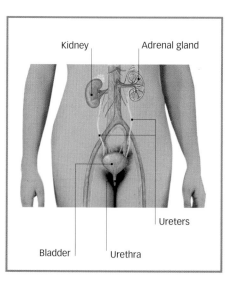

Kidney

Adrenal gland

Ureters

Bladder

Urethra

DO YOUR DAILY KEGELS

During the late 1940s, Dr Arnold Kegel, a University of California surgeon, designed a special exercise to help women who complained of leaking urine. This exercise – now known as 'Kegels' – helps to strengthen the pubococcygeal (PC) muscle, which supports the bladder and urethra. This is the muscle that you use to stop the flow of urine in midstream, or to 'hold back' on a bowel movement. It is important to keep your PC muscle strong during your menopausal years to avoid potential bladder control problems.

A well-toned PC muscle can also contribute to increased sexual satisfaction, as this is the muscle that you can feel contracting rhythmically during orgasm.

To do your Kegels, think of your pelvic floor as a lift in a five-storey building:

- Slowly tighten the PC muscle, imagining that the lift is moving up floor by floor.
- At each floor, count to five before tightening the muscle further.
- When you reach the top, go down floor by floor again, relaxing your PC muscle gradually as you go.
- Try to do at least five Kegels in a row, several times a day. They can be done anytime, anywhere: at your desk at work, while waiting in line at the supermarket, while watching television or even while making love.

Osteoporosis

The skeleton is a living thing which is continually renewing itself with new bone. Bone constantly undergoes breakdown and renewal in a controlled process necessary for bone growth and repair. This process is known as re-modelling.

The basic structure of your bones will not change with age, but their density and strength will reduce. This is part of the natural ageing process for men as well as women, but for some of us, the bone will be lost much faster than new bone can be formed to replace it. If this happens, bones can become so fragile that they are liable to break very easily: fractures commonly occur at the wrist, hip and spine,

This fractured bone has jagged edges. Consequently, it will take time for it to knit together.

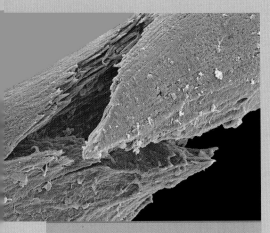

and the consequences can be devastating with about 20 per cent of hip fractures resulting in death.

The condition known as osteoporosis is a worldwide disease, as evidenced by the formation of support, information and research organizations for osteoporosis in 70 countries. Racial origin influences a woman's risk of brittle bones – women of African, Aboriginal or Mediterranean extraction are unlikely to suffer osteopororis because they usually possess thicker bones and have reached a greater bone mass at skeletal maturity. On the other hand, Caucasian, Asian or Oriental women possess generally thinner bones and lower bone mass, and therefore face a greater risk.

Osteoporosis can begin anywhere from 5 to 20 years before the menopause when oestrogen levels are still high. It accelerates for a few years at the menopause or if the ovaries are surgically removed or become non-functioning, as can happen after a hysterectomy. At such times, the rate of bone loss will increase from 2 to 5 per cent a year. However, for some women its foundations may well have been laid many years earlier by a diet grossly deficient in calcium, or a demanding athletic schedule which inhibited ovulation.

Osteoporosis is a silent disease which goes unnoticed and is usually painless in the early stages. Because you cannot see your bones, you may not know there is anything amiss until you break your hip, spine or wrist due to a minor bump or fall. Other symptoms include:

- loss in height
- a curving spine
- acute and unexplained back pain.

Osteoporosis can lead to a dramatic loss of height, severe curvature of the spine, chronic pain and permanent disability. It can literally devastate lives, and everyday activities that we all take for granted can become impossible.

RISK FACTORS

The following place you at high risk of suffering from osteoporosis:

- Very early menopause before the age of 45 – this causes early loss of oestrogen because your ovaries stop working.
- An early menopause before the normal age of 50 – early loss of oestrogen is likely, and certain if your ovaries are removed.
- Long-term use of high-dose corticosteroids (for conditions such as arthritis and asthma). Do not stop taking them – your doctor may be able to adjust your dosage to compensate for bone loss.
- Irregular or infrequent menstruation – this can happen naturally or be caused by over-exercising, if you are a dancer, or suffer from anorexia nervosa or bulimia. This results in low oestrogen levels similar to menopause, regardless of age.
- Disorders of the digestion that cause malabsorption problems, such as coeliac disease, Crohn's disease or gastric surgery.
- Smoking – this can damage bone-building cells and cause an early menopause.
- Low calcium intake – consumption of milk and dairy products maintains bone density.

I began suffering severe back pain in 1995, and thought it was just the 'ageing' effect. But as time went on, my agility and mobility plummeted, and I had to depend more and more on my family for help. Visits to the doctor led to pain killers, then stronger pain killers, and I lost three precious years before I was found to have suffered severe loss of bone density.

CARMEN (Spain)

- Heavy drinking – alcohol abuse can cause bone to deteriorate.
- Immobility – bones need exercise to remain strong, so those who are bed- and wheelchair-bound are more at risk.
- Lack of sunshine – exposure to sunlight is necessary for the production of vitamin D which is essential for bone health as a bone hardener.

Much of the variation in bone mineral mass and the incidence of osteoporosis can be ascribed to genetic differences between individuals, and therefore a family history of osteoporosis puts you more at risk of having fractures later in life. If you are aware of a history of osteoporosis in your family, you would be well advised to ask your doctor about bone density testing.

DRINK MORE MILK

In 1994, a cross-sectional study of 284 women aged 44–74 living in Cambridge, UK, revealed that frequent milk consumption before the age of 25 was associated with 5 per cent higher hip-bone mineral density in middle-aged and older women.

DID YOU KNOW?

A child's skeleton is replaced every two years, an adult's every 7–10 years. After bones have stopped growing in length at the age of 16–18 years, they still increase in density. After about the age of 35 years they begin to deteriorate.

DIAGNOSIS

The best way to identify osteoporosis in its early form is a test using X-rays called dual energy X-ray absorptiometry (DXA), often referred to as a DXA scan. This can detect tiny amounts of bone loss of 1–3 per cent and regular yearly scans allow the rate of loss to be calculated.

At present, this method of bone density scanning is the most accurate and reliable method of assessing the strength of your bones. A DXA machine will usually scan your lower spine and one hip. Other areas that can also be assessed include your forearm and heel. Your bone density is then compared to young, healthy adult measurements.

DXA machines are large, static pieces of

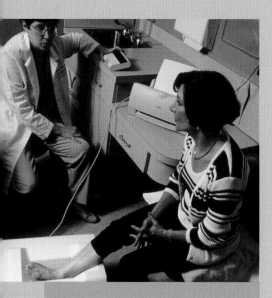

BONE DENSITY TESTING
Whatever is used to predict osteoporotic fractures, a measure of bone mass is only valuable if associated with a clinical comment and opinion from a registered medical doctor experienced in bone mass measurement.

equipment. A less expensive diagnostic method uses a portable ultrasound machine which can assess your bone structure and strength, usually of your heel bone (calcaneus), wrist or finger. Heel ultrasound is also useful in predicting your osteoporotic fracture risk around the time of your menopause and your Colles (wrist) fracture risk in the early post-menopausal years.

REDUCE YOUR RISK BY INVESTING IN YOUR BONES

Calcium accounts for approximately 67 per cent of bone weight and bones act as a storage bank for calcium. If the amount of calcium in your blood falls below a certain level, your body will take its calcium needs from your bones. This calcium withdrawn from your bones is used for other important functions of your body carried out by the heart, muscles, blood and nerves.

Clearly, it is important to maintain your intake of dietary calcium and the chart opposite sets out ways in which you can increase this. However, it is also important to be aware of the way that other substances in foods and drinks can affect your calcium levels.

Substances that can reduce calcium absorption (when taken in large quantities) include the following:

- Phytates – present in fibre, particularly unprocessed bran
- Tannins – present in tea
- Oxalate – present in spinach
- Caffeine – present in coffee, tea and cola drinks
- Phosphates without calcium – present in fizzy, canned drinks

Increasing your calcium intake

Daily requirement
before menopause 1,000 mg
after menopause 1,500 mg

Calcium content of common foods in milligrams per 100 g (approx 3½ oz) of food

DAIRY

Cheese	
Cheddar	800
Cottage	80
Danish blue	580
Edam	740
Parmesan	1,220
Processed	700
Spread	510
Cream	79
Egg (whole)	52
Egg (yolk)	130
Milk (semi-skimmed)	
0.5 litre (1 pint)	702
Milk (skimmed)	
0.5 litre (1 pint)	705
Yogurt – low fat	180
Ice cream	134

VEGETABLES

Beans, haricot	180
Beans, kidney	140
Broccoli	100
Cabbage	53
Chick peas	140
Greens – kale	98
Olives in brine	61
Parsley	330
Peas	31
Spinach	600
Spring onions	140
Watercress	220
Baked potato (large)	24
Baked beans	
(350 g/12¼ oz can)	239

MEAT AND FISH

Meat and fish contain very small amounts of calcium. Most pies and fish in batter contain calcium in the flour. Canned pilchards and sardines, sprats and whitebait contain calcium in the bones.

Prawns	150
Crab (canned)	120
Pilchards (canned)	300
Salmon (canned)	93
Sardines (canned)	460–550
Sprats (fried)	620–710
Whitebait (fried)	860
Fish paste	280
Steamed scallops	120

FRUIT

Apricots, dried	92
Blackcurrants	60
Currants	95
Figs	280
Lemon, whole	110
Rhubarb	100
Orange (1 large)	99

NUTS AND SEEDS

Almonds	250
Brazils	180
Peanuts, roasted and	
salted	61
Sesame seeds	870

DRINKS (DRY WEIGHT)

Cocoa powder	130
Coffee, ground	130
instant	160
Malted milk drink	230
Tea, Indian	430

FLOUR AND BAKED FOODS

Bread, white or brown	100
Cake, sponge	140
rock (individual fruit cake)	390
Flour, plain	210–40
self-raising	350
Soya flour	210–40
Wheat bran	110

COOKING INGREDIENTS

Curry powder	640
Mustard, dry	330
Pepper	130
Salt	230
Stock cubes	180
Yeast, dried	80

Substances that increase the loss of calcium in your urine include:

- Salt – a high salt intake increases urinary calcium loss
- Protein – excessive intake (more than four times a day) of protein derived from animal sources
- Caffeine – coffee, tea and other caffeine-containing drinks cause increased output of urine, therefore increased loss of calcium

Your bones need vitamin D

Vitamin D enhances calcium absorption. It is present in apples, watercress, tuna, salmon and herring. But the best source of vitamin D is sunlight which increases vitamin D production in the skin.

Your bones need magnesium

Magnesium is essential for the proper metabolism of calcium, and your bones need twice as much magnesium as calcium if the biochemistry of your bone formation is to run smoothly. Good sources are dark green vegetables, apples, seeds, nuts, figs and lemons, as well as whole grains such as brown rice, whole wheat and whole rye.

Your bones need vitamins C, B6 and K

Vitamin C is crucial for bone formation as it produces collagen (fibrous matter) which makes up some 90 per cent of the bone matrix. Good sources of vitamin C include citrus fruits (oranges, lemons, limes), green and leafy vegetables, berries, potatoes, sweet potatoes and yams.

Vitamin B6 appears to increase the strength of connective tissue in bones. It is found in wholegrains, fish, nuts, bananas and avocados.

Vitamin K is known primarily for its effect on blood clotting and it helps to harden bone – the best source is green vegetables.

Your bones need exercise

The best type of exercise to strengthen bones is weight-bearing exercise. Your bones need to be loaded as you move. Good weight-bearing exercises include walking, jumping, ice-skating, running, skipping, ball sports, running up and down stairs, digging the garden, aerobics and tennis. You need to aim to exercise for 20 minutes a day, three times a week.

WHAT ELSE CAN BE DONE?
Taking dietary supplements can help to increase the amount of vitamins and minerals that your body receives each day.

DID YOU KNOW?
Gardening boosts self-esteem, builds confidence and will soon be prescribed by doctors.

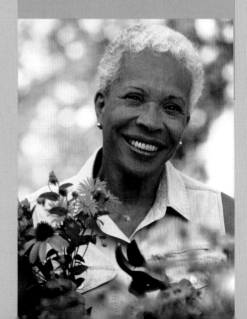

> " *My mother is only 69 years old, yet she has a hunchback (kyphosis) that results in severe back pain which prevents her sitting for long periods of time. She has lost 6cm in height, has problems finding suitable clothing and can wear only sports shoes to prevent possible falls. She was diagnosed as suffering from severe osteoporosis nearly 20 years after the onset of her menopause. I am not taking any chances – I take daily calcium supplements, and undergo bone density testing every two years.*
>
> SARAH (Israel) "

In this picture you can clearly see the effects of osteoporosis on the spine.

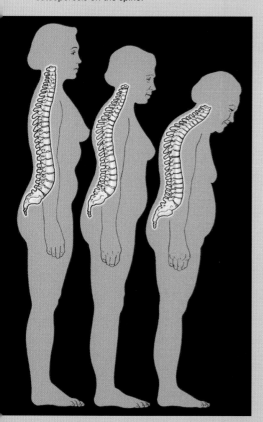

Calcium supplements

These may be advisable if you cannot obtain your recommended daily intake through food and drink (see the chart on page 35 for the calcium content of common foods).

Vitamin D and calcitonins

Vitamin D supplements are recommended for people with vitamin D deficiency as a result of poor diet or limited exposure to sunlight, for example if you are aged over 65 and housebound or living in an institution. Remember, however, that excessive exposure to sun can cause skin cancer.

Calcitrol (trade names Rocaltrol and Calcijex) helps to increase the amount of calcium absorption in the gut and the amount of calcium that enters the bone.

FALLS AND THEIR PREVENTION

Most of the fractures associated with osteoporosis are caused by falls. A third of people over the age of 60 have a fall at least once a year and although not all falls are serious, many result in fractures, especially in older women with osteoporosis.

The chart below describes some of the most common reasons for falls and provides suggestions for ways to prevent such falls.

WHO IS AT RISK?

Most hip fractures occur in people aged over 80 years, with associated high morbidity and mortality. It is therefore desirable to identify those individuals who are at greatest risk, because that risk can be roughly halved with effective treatment.

Ignac Fogelman, Professor of Nuclear Medicine, Guy's Hospital, London

COMMON REASONS FOR FALLS

Reasons	Prevention
Poor balance caused by weak muscles, low blood pressure, ear problems or other conditions	• *Exercise keeps muscles strong and improves balance*
Poor eyesight, making it harder to notice hazards such as a trailing cord or a bump in the footpath	• *Make sure you have good lighting in your home* • *Get an annual eye test* • *Avoid glare by wearing good-quality sunglasses*
Footwear	• *Ensure your shoes are well-fitting*
Hazards at home (most falls occur in the home)	• *Floor surfaces – mats, carpets, rugs should lie flat without curled-up edges* • *Make sure electrical cords are not hanging where you walk*
Lighting	• *Have clear lighting in all areas in your home with easily accessible switches*
Bathroom	• *Have hand rails fitted to help you in/out of the shower/bathtub and when using the toilet* • *Use non-slip mats to avoid slippery wet surfaces*
Hazards outside the home	• *Be aware of uneven pavements, slippery shopping centre floors, steep kerbs and so on* • *Keep your garden free of clutter including fallen branches and hosepipes*

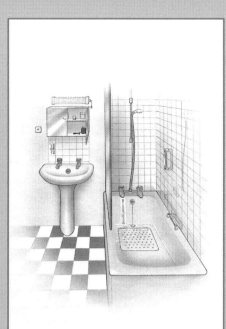

BATHROOM SAFETY

There are some simple precautions you can take to avoid falls in the bathroom. Install hand rails for getting in and out of the bath and always use a non-slip bathmat.

SUMMARY

If you have experienced an early menopause – prolonged amenorrhea (abnormal suppression or absence of menstruation other than because of pregnancy); if you have a family history of osteoporosis or are taking corticosteroids, then a bone scan will be helpful in reaching a decision about treatment. Explore all your options for maintaining healthy bones for the rest of your life – if you care for your bones, then your bones will take care of you.

" At the age of 49 I had a full hysterectomy as a result of cancer. In my late 50s I broke several ribs falling over a box, and broke several others ten years later. Then in 1995, at the age of 63, I fell off a ladder and broke a leg, fractured my sternum, cracked my collar-bone, chipped an elbow and again broke four ribs. It was only then that I was diagnosed with osteoporosis, when a bone density scan showed I was at extreme risk of fracture of my hips and spine.

My doctor put me on a programme of daily medication to build up my bone mass which I've kept up for the last four years. Even so, my bones are still extremely brittle: last week when bringing in the groceries from the car, I used my little finger to lift a plastic supermarket bag containing two 1-litre cartons of milk and my finger snapped.

For me, living with osteoporosis means:

- *I must be careful all the time.*
- *I must not hurry, especially on uneven surfaces and on rainy days.*
- *I must keep my dog on a short leash when I walk her each day so that I don't get tangled up and trip over.*
- *I must not wear high heels.*
- *Because of its effects on bone density, I must limit alcohol or, better still, abstain.*
- *I must carry in groceries in small amounts, making several trips up 17 stairs.*
- *I must no longer dig the vegetable garden or climb or stretch up to trim trees.*
- *I must only spring clean things I can reach from floor level.*

Most of all, it means not being able to run around with my grandchildren – I'm the person sitting on the beach minding the shoes, instead of exploring the rockpools.

BONNIE (New Zealand)

"

Breast awareness

As you grow older it becomes increasingly important to be aware of the health of your breasts. Breast cancer is a disease that affected over a million people worldwide in the year 2000, one-third of whom lived in Europe. About 60 per cent of breast cancers occur in women over the age of 60 and the risk is greatest after the age of 75.

SELF-EXAMINATION

It is important to know how to check your breasts yourself.

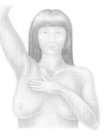

Check each breast for lumps, differences in skin texture and changes around the nipple. Feel right into each armpit.

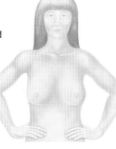

Repeat this check in several positions and with your arms in different postures.

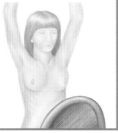

Try standing in front of a mirror to help you become more familiar with your breasts.

THE WAY FORWARD FOR YOU

Although it is impossible, at present, to predict who will develop breast cancer, you have a higher risk if you:

- have a strong family history of breast cancer
- carry a breast cancer gene
- started your periods early (aged 10 or under) and have a late (aged 59 plus) menopause
- have no children or have them late in life (aged over 40)
- have a history of benign breast disease.

Unfortunately, you cannot do anything about most of the above, apart from being aware of them. But you can make sure you that you examine your breasts regularly and go for screening tests known as mammograms.

Breast cancer and oestrogen

The contraceptive Pill contains oestrogen, which can stimulate cancer cells to grow. In theory, increasing the supply of oestrogen could trigger a breast cancer to develop – in practice, the risk of this happening appears to be a small one. Recent research looking at the contraceptive Pill worldwide has revealed that:

- the incidence of breast cancer is increased slightly while the Pill is taken and for up to 10 years after stopping
- more than 10 years after stopping the risk is the same as that of a woman who has never taken it
- a large number of women diagnosed with breast cancer have used the contraceptive Pill during the progression of their malignant disease process.

Breast cancer and diet

So far, the search for dietary factors implicated in breast cancer during adulthood has been disappointing. This does not preclude a possible association between breast cancer and diet earlier in life. The only fairly well-established dietary risk for breast cancer is alcohol – a small but consistent increase in risk has been associated with alcohol consumption.

Strong family history

If your mother, sister or daughter was diagnosed with breast cancer under the age of 40 years, or if you have two or more relatives diagnosed (both from one side of your family), at least one of whom is under 50 years old, or if several relatives on the same side of your family have developed breast, ovarian or colon cancer, then you have what is known as a strong family history.

This may indicate that there is a breast cancer gene in your family. Several genes have been identified that can increase breast cancer risk, but at present there are tests for only two of them: BRCA1 and BRCA2. Your risk of getting breast cancer if you carry either of these genes is about 85 per cent by the time you are 55 years old. In other words, 85 women out of 100 who carry a breast cancer gene will develop breast cancer by the time they are 55.

Benign breast disease

If you have a history of benign breast lumps, then you are at a very slightly increased risk of breast cancer. But 'benign breast disease' includes a wide range of different conditions, most of which do not lead to cancer. One in ten breast lumps show 'atypical hyperplasia'. This means that the cells are not cancerous, but they are growing abnormally, and will increase your risk of breast cancer by up to four times the average.

SUMMARY

Although many of the risk factors for breast cancer are beyond your control, you can still take steps to decrease your risk by reducing your alcohol consumption and eating more fresh fruit, bran cereals, wholemeal bread and raw salads daily.

The earlier that breast cancer is detected, the more effectively it can be treated. This is why it is essential to examine your breasts regularly and make sure you attend mammogram appointments.

Regular mammograms offer reassurance to women as potentially cancerous changes can be detected at an early stage.

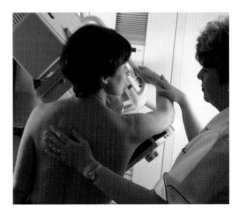

Alzheimer's disease

Alzheimer's disease (also called pre-senile dementia) was named after a German doctor, Alois Alzheimer (1864–1915). He published many papers on conditions and diseases of the brain, one of which involved memory loss, behaviour and personality changes as well as a decline in cognitive abilities.

These clinical definitions in no way convey the pain and heartbreak experienced if you are intimately involved with someone who develops the disease. The actual degenerative process begins in mid-life and is almost impossible to reverse.

RISK FACTORS

You are at increased risk of developing Alzheimer's disease if you have high blood pressure and/or high levels of cholesterol (see page 44) or if one of your parents or grandparents suffered from it.

One theory is that you may be at extra risk if you undergo a dramatic loss of oestrogen at menopause, as evidenced by symptoms including memory lapses and erratic concentration. Given that the hypothalamus at the base of the brain acts as a control centre for your hormones, it would seem logical to assume that a major hormonal disturbance would be bound to have an effect on the brain.

REDUCING THE RISK

There is promising evidence that the herbal supplement gingko biloba is effective in improving memory. A review of 33 clinical trials of the herb, dating back to 1976, suggests that it has a role to play in enhancing brain function.

Consult your doctor about taking gingko biloba as it may interact with other drugs.

Particular care must be taken if you are on anticoagulant therapy – for example, Warfarin or aspirin – or if you suffer with blood clotting.

SUMMARY

Neither dementia nor Alzheimer's disease is necessarily part of the ageing process. It is therefore very important to consider the implications for you if your family medical history includes either of them, especially if you have high blood pressure and/or high levels of cholesterol.

I was very alarmed when my mother was menopausal in her 50s. She forgot where things belonged, like once putting a bottle of milk in the oven, muddled up her words and couldn't remember the names of her grandchildren. Her anxiety levels soared because of all this and her moods were dreadful. Thankfully, she changed back to her old self after she took gingko biloba regularly for about six months.

REBECCA (Oxford)

Keeping your mind active delays the onset of problems with memory recall.

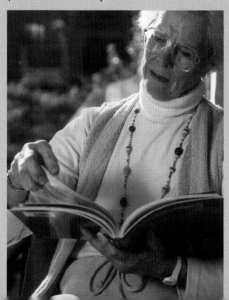

Bowel cancer

Nearly a million people were diagnosed with bowel cancer worldwide in the year 2000, of whom just under one-third live in Europe.

Bowel cancer is the third commonest cancer in the UK (after lung and breast cancer) and the second leading cause of all cancer death in the USA. Nine out of ten cancers of the colon and rectum develop because of sporadic mutations in the cells lining the bowel. Sporadic mutations, which happen at random, accumulate over time and are caused by diet and the effects of advancing age.

RISK FACTORS

One of the risk factors is a family history of the disease. Certain criteria indicating a pattern of bowel cancer throughout generations can be evaluated using the Amsterdam Criteria. These state that a person's risk of developing bowel cancer is high if their family includes:

- three members with colon or rectal cancer
- at least two successive generations with colon or rectal cancer
- two family members with the disease who are first-degree relatives (parents, brothers, sisters or children) of another family member with colon and rectal cancer
- at least one member affected at or before the age of 50.

Over the last 20 years, death rates from this disease have dropped more in women than in men, and evidence suggests that post-menopausal hormone use may reduce the risk.

SUMMARY

- You need to consider the implications for you if your family medical history indicates you are at risk of this cancer.
- Improving and modifying your eating lifestyle will be of benefit.

WHERE DOES BOWEL CANCER DEVELOP?

Bowel cancer usually affects the last part of the large intestine and the rectum.

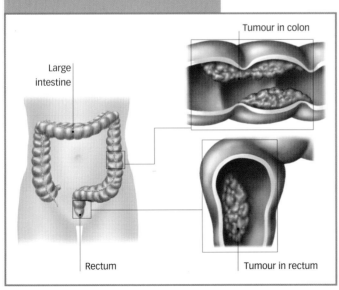

Large intestine

Tumour in colon

Rectum

Tumour in rectum

THE PARADOX
The risk of bowel cancer in pre-menopausal women is doubled if they are clinically obese, although after the menopause the fat tissue is an important source of oestrogen which may reduce the risk of colo-rectal cancer.

Heart disease

If you hold out your hand, palm upwards, you will see bluish veins visible under the fine skin of your wrist – these are part of an intricate vascular system circulating blood throughout your body.

High blood pressure Blood pressure means the pressure of the blood in your arteries – the tubes that take blood away from your heart to the rest of your body. High blood pressure happens if the walls of the larger arteries lose their elasticity and become rigid, and the smaller vessels contract (become narrower). People with high blood pressure run a higher risk of suffering a stroke or heart attack.

Peripheral arterial disease This happens when the arteries that supply blood to the legs become narrowed or completely blocked off. Other arteries, such as those supplying blood to the heart and neck, are also likely to be affected.

Diabetes and heart disease These are two of the world's most common chronic diseases. More than 10 million people in Europe suffer from diabetes.

Blood cholesterol There are two types of cholesterol: dietary and blood. Dietary is contained in food, while blood cholesterol is the amount circulating in the body. Cholesterol is manufactured in the liver and can be deposited in the artery walls by a process called atherosclerosis, which leads to narrowing and hardening of the arteries and then to heart disease.

A healthy blood supply flows freely, but sometimes blockages can occur (as in a blood clot) or the veins become furred up (like the inside of a kettle) and if one of these happens to you, you are at risk of suffering either a stroke or a heart attack. These two conditions are part of the group of disorders known as cardiovascular disease (CVD).

CVD includes all diseases of the heart and blood vessels. The two main diseases in this category are coronary heart disease (CHD) and stroke, but CVD also includes congenital heart disease (heart deformities present at birth), valvular heart disease, and a range of other diseases of the heart and blood vessels. Both CHD and stroke have a similar cause – a blockage in an artery.

Coronary heart disease (CHD) comes in two main forms: angina and heart attack – the latter is also known as a myocardial infarction.

- Angina is caused by a narrowing of the blood vessels to the heart muscle. It is experienced as a pain in the chest brought on by exercise or emotion. It can be mild or severe and generally lasts for less than 10 minutes.
- A heart attack causes similar pain but lasts longer and can be fatal. A heart attack results when a blood vessel is entirely blocked by a blood clot.

Cardiovascular disease is a more common cause of morbidity and mortality for women in most countries of the world than osteoporosis and cancer combined. However, it is unusual for cardio-vascular events to occur before women are in their 60s.

RISK FACTORS

The following factors place you at high risk of CVD (cardiovascular disease):

- High blood pressure – the most important risk factor for a stroke
- A family history of heart disease
- Obesity – this is defined as having a body mass index (BMI) of 30 or higher. A BMI of 26 or higher classifies you as overweight (see the formula for measuring your BMI on page 47)
- A sedentary lifestyle
- Cigarette smoking – consistently associated with peripheral arterial disease
- Psychosocial factors – stressful situations, depression and social isolation have been linked to increased risk
- Diabetes
- High blood cholesterol – associated with cardiovascular disease

The combined effect of two or more risk factors is more powerful than any one risk factor, and some risk factors commonly occur together. For example, screening for diabetes may be appropriate in women who have high blood pressure.

THE HEART OF THE MATTER

As we get older, our pattern of risk changes. On average, women acquire heart disease about ten years later than men. Coronary heart disease rates become more similar in men and women as they age but this reflects a deceleration in male rates of heart disease during middle age, rather than an acceleration in women's post-menopausal rates.

DID YOU KNOW?

Every year, more than 500,000 people die in the European Union as a result of using tobacco, with an average loss of 21 years in life expectancy.

BLOCKED ARTERIES

The process of coronary heart disease (CHD) begins when the coronary arteries become narrowed by a gradual build-up of fatty material (atheroma) within their walls.

High blood pressure or high cholesterol levels in mid life, and in particular the combination of these risks, increases the risk of Alzheimer's disease in later life by inducing atherosclerosis and impairing blood flow to the brain.

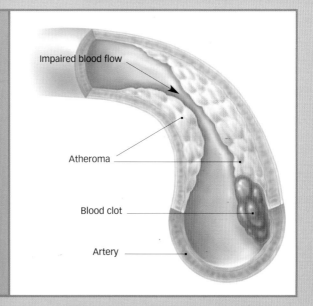

Impaired blood flow

Atheroma

Blood clot

Artery

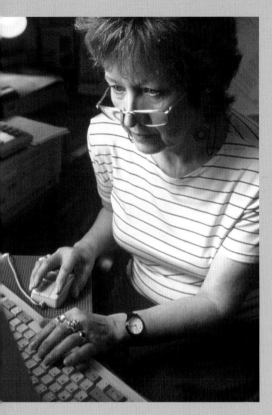

A sedentary lifestyle can place you at risk of heart disease. If your job requires you to sit at a desk all day, then make sure that the rest of your life isn't so sedentary.

diagnosed, so that comparatively little is known about it. For years it has been assumed that women are protected from heart disease as long as oestrogen is produced, because this has a beneficial effect on blood cholesterol metabolism. It therefore followed that women lost that protection after the menopause because of the loss of oestrogen, hence the increased risk.

As discussed in Chapter 1, women do indeed lose oestrogen during the menopausal years – approximately 40 per cent of it – but it continues to be produced in variable quantities for up to 20 years after the menopause.

The observation that the progression of CVD in women is more rapid after the menopause led to the hypothesis that maintaining oestrogen levels with HRT could prevent it. Indeed, since the 1970s, more than 30 case-control and prospective studies have reported less heart disease in women using oestrogen.

However, one meta-analysis of 22 randomized trials before 1997 that compared HRT with placebo, no therapy or vitamins/minerals in predominantly healthy post-menopausal women showed no overall cardioprotective effect of HRT.

A huge amount of research has been conducted on men and heart disease, but CVD in women is under-researched and under-

CVD IS LARGELY PREVENTABLE

This has been successfuly demonstrated by a community-wide heart health programme carried out in the Finnish region of North Karelia, where over a period of 20 years CVD mortality fell by around 70 per cent.

TOO MANY BROKEN HEARTS

CVD accounts for more than half of all deaths in Europe of people aged under 75, with a total of four million lives taken every year. The Greeks smoke the most and have the biggest problem with CVD; the Portuguese exercise the least and have the highest death rate in the EU from stroke; the Irish are the most likely nationality to die from coronary heart disease (CHD).

Body mass index

The amount of body fat you carry may be more significant than your weight alone. The Body Mass Index (BMI) expresses the relationship between a person's weight and height. It is calculated as weight in kilograms, divided by height in metres squared. The best way to determine a good weight range for you is to use the BMI formula – you will find a calculator helpful in working it out. Your BMI should fall somewhere between 18 and 25. To be either below 18 or above 25 is to put your health at risk.

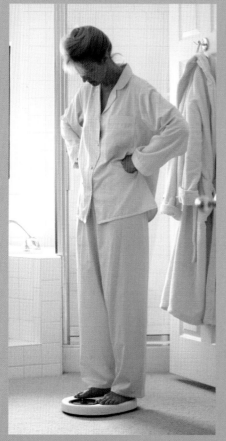

CALCULATING YOUR BODY MASS INDEX

Here are 2 ways to work out your BMI:

Method 1
1 Your weight (in kilograms) is X.
2 Multiply your height (in metres) by your height (in metres). This is Y.
3 Divide X by Y.

Method 2
1 Multiply your present weight (in pounds) by 704. This is X.
2 Multiply your height (in inches) by your height (in inches). This is Y.
3 Divide X by Y.

Example
Let's say you are 5 feet 4 in (64 in) tall and weigh 142 lb.

Multiply 142 by 704 – this totals 99,968.

Next, multiply 64 by 64 for a total of 4,096.

Divide 99,968 by 4,096 to result in a BMI of around 24.

You are within a healthy range, although near the high end, and you should be aware that if you gain 10 lb, your BMI will be in the unhealthy range.

Watch your weight during this menopausal transition, as any excess could affect your heart.

BLOOD CLOTS

When your arteries are blocked by fatty deposits, blood cannot flow freely and there is an increased likelihood of blood clots forming. If a blood clot forms in the coronary artery, blood cannot get to your heart and the result is a heart attack. If a blood clot occurs in your brain, the result is a stroke. The risk factors for a blood clot are:

- a personal or family history of venous thromboembolism (blood clots)
- recent surgery or trauma
- obesity
- severe varicose veins
- prolonged immobilization.

Although some of these risk factors are beyond your control, you can diminish the risk of blood clots developing by becoming active soon after you have had surgery, losing weight if you are obese and seeking medical help if you have varicose veins.

REDUCING YOUR RISK

There are many dietary and lifestyle changes that you can make to reduce your risk of cardiovascular disease:

- Include more oily fish, nuts, seeds and oils in your meals. The essential fatty acids in these foods are important for the prevention of heart disease. Eating fish three times a week reduces the risk of CVD as fish oils lower cholesterol, thin your blood and reduce the risk of narrowing of the arteries.
- Try to stay within an appropriate weight range for your height and frame.
- Stop smoking cigarettes and avoid 'passive' smoking situations.

VITAMIN E

A study by scientists at Cambridge University and Papworth Hospital, UK, in 1996 found that a daily dose of vitamin E reduced the risk of having a heart attack by 75 per cent. This 18-month double-blind controlled trial involved 2,000 patients with coronary atherosclerosis (see box, page 45). The number of heart attacks in the group taking the vitamin E was a quarter of that in the group taking placebo.

If you smoke you are more at risk of heart disease.

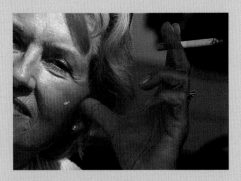

- Eat more soya. Soya beans are a complete protein as they contain all eight essential amino acids.
- Eat more fresh vegetables and fruit as well as dried fruit. Fibre in potatoes, carrots, apples, beans and oats binds up the cholesterol and carries it out of your body.
- Take vitamin E supplements.
- If you have a disability that prevents you from taking active exercise, try to arrange regular physiotherapy, massage and hydrotherapy sessions.

ISCHAEMIC HEART DISEASE

'Ischaemia' means an inadequate supply of blood, and is a consequence of the gradual narrowing of the coronary arteries that supply blood and oxygen to the muscles of the heart.

SUMMARY

Be aware of the risk factors for heart disease. Help keep your heart and blood vessels healthy by:

- eliminating two or more of your risk factors
- improving your lifestyle and adopting healthier eating habits
- taking regular weight-bearing exercise.

You can maintain muscle mass with these handheld weights by training for at least 1 hour a week.

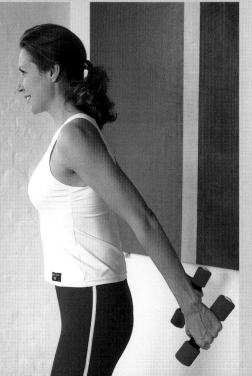

RAW FOOD FOR A HEALTHY HEART

An ambitious study between 1973 and 1979 recruited 11,000 British men and women from among the customers of health food shops and other people with an interest in health foods and vegetarianism.

Its aim was to examine the relationship between six dietary factors – a vegetarian diet and consumption of wholemeal bread, bran cereals, nuts and dried fruit, fresh fruit and raw salad – and mortality for which associations with diet have been suggested.

The most significant association revealed after a 17-year follow-up to 1995 that daily consumption of raw salad was associated with a 26 per cent reduction in death from ischaemic heart disease (see box, above left), slightly greater than that for fresh fruit (24 per cent).

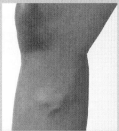

Severe varicose veins are a predisposing factor in the risk of developing a blood clot.

DID YOU KNOW?

One clinical trial showed that a 'Mediterranean diet' supplemented with alpha-linoleic acid found in seeds and nuts significantly reduced the risk of recurrent coronary events in patients with heart disease.

The special case of diabetes

Diabetes is one of the world's two most common chronic diseases, and more than 10 million people in Europe have the disease. Diabetic women are at greatly increased risk of developing ischaemic heart disease (see box, page 49).

Diabetes mellitis is a condition in which the amount of glucose (sugar) in the blood is too high because the sufferer's body cannot use it properly.

Glucose comes from the digestion of starchy foods such as bread, rice, potatoes, chapatis, yams and plantain, as well as sugar and other sweet foods. It is also produced in the body in the liver.

THE TWO TYPES OF DIABETES

There are two main types of diabetes:

- Type 1 diabetes, also known as insulin-dependent diabetes, usually appears before the age of 40.
- Type 2 diabetes, also known as non-insulin-dependent diabetes, is more common among women after, rather than prior to, the menopause.

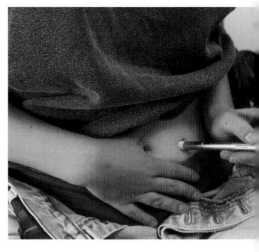

Type 1 diabetes is treated by insulin injections, but you may not need injections if you suffer from Type 2 diabetes.

Type 1 diabetes develops if the body is unable to produce any insulin (a hormone produced by the pancreas) and it is treated by insulin injections. Dietary changes are essential. Type 2 diabetes (late onset, in mid-life or older) develops when the body can still produce some insulin but not enough, or when the insulin that is produced does not work properly. It is treated either by diet and exercise alone; by diet, exercise and tablets; or by diet, exercise and insulin injections.

The risk of death from cardiovascular disease (CVD) is five times greater in women aged 50–60 years who have diabetes than in women of the same age who do not. Coronary heart disease (CHD) is a major cause of morbidity and mortality in post-menopausal women with Type 2 diabetes. Furthermore, the Framingham Study (a long-term American health research project begun in 1948) showed a sixfold increase of sudden cardiac death in female compared with male diabetic patients.

DIABETES AND OSTEOPOROSIS

Women with Type 1 diabetes have reduced bone density, which can be demonstrated after a few years of insulin treatment. While it is known that insulin is important for the growth of bone cells and mineral metabolism, the exact mechanism of the osteopenia of diabetes is not fully understood.

Type 2 diabetic women have increased bone turnover but normal bone density.

If you have Type 2 diabetes, other members of your family may also be at risk, particularly if they:

- are overweight
- are aged between 40–75 years
- are of Asian or Afro-Caribbean origin
- have a history of gestational diabetes (diabetes in pregnancy).

A WEIGHTY PROBLEM

Research data from over 44,000 people with Type 2 diabetes was presented at a recent Diabetes UK medical conference. It revealed that not only do diabetics have a higher risk of serious complications and premature death, but that obesity makes the situation worse.

As many as 80 per cent of people are overweight when they are diagnosed with Type 2 diabetes, and this obesity could be reducing their life expectancy by up to eight years. Losing weight helps to:

- control blood glucose levels by reducing the body's resistance to insulin
- lower blood fats like cholestrol
- lower blood pressure
- reduce the risk of heart disease and stroke.

Making changes to your eating habits

There are several ways in which you can make quick and effective changes to your diet:

- Look at your plate: you may need to eat less food as well as change the proportions of food on your plate.
- Cut down on fat. Grill, bake, microwave or poach foods without any added fat or oil. Choose low-fat dairy products such as skimmed or semi-skimmed milk, low-fat

yogurt and reduced-fat cheese. Look out for unsalted versions of spreads and fats to reduce your sodium intake. Use oils and spreads that are high in monunsaturated fats (olive oil, rapeseed oil and nut oils) or polyunsaturated fats (sunflower, safflower, soya, corn or grapeseed oils).
- Eat more fruit and vegetables. Aim to eat at least five portions of fruit and vegetables every day. Make vegetables or salad the largest serving on your plate.
- Include some starchy foods like bread, potatoes, chapatis, rice, cereals or pasta at each meal. Wholegrain cereals, bread and other wholewheat products are more filling than white versions.
- Don't skip meals to lose weight. Eating regular meals helps control appetite as well as blood sugar levels.
- Look at your snacks. Fruit makes an ideal snack in place of crisps, biscuits, chocolate, cakes or pastries.
- Alcohol is high in calories and stimulates your appetite. Aim to cut down.

HEALTH ON THE SHELF

Raised blood glucose reduces absorption of nutrients and enhances their excretion, hence there are indications of deficiencies of magnesium, zinc and chromium in people suffering from diabetes.

In one recent UK study, 27 people with Type 2 diabetes (controlled by diet and tablets) reported greater vitality and less anxiety after undergoing three months of daily multi-nutrient supplementation.

Stress – and how to live with it comfortably

Psychosocial factors – life stress situations, depression and social isolation – have been linked to increased risk of cardiovascular disease (pages 44–49). Whatever you do in your daily life and whatever your circumstances, you will encounter stress every day. It is part of the human condition begun even before birth, for even a baby can show signs of distress in its mother's womb.

Stress is a catalyst for change as it provides us with excitement, stimulation and motivation. But it can accelerate to dangerous levels, which can damage our health. All of us need to learn effective ways of coping with stress, as

- high levels of emotional stress increase susceptibility to illness
- chronic stress results in a suppression of our immune systems, which in turn increases our susceptibility to illness
- emotional stress also suppresses our immune systems and can lead to hormonal imbalances.

It would be reassuring if at least our menopausal years were ones of contentment where a calmer, less frenetic pace replaced years of pressure. All too often this does not happen, because we allow ourselves to feel powerless in the face of the demands, needs and expectations of other people, frequently as a consequence of our own lack of self-esteem.

In over 20 years' work as a counsellor, I have talked with hundreds of anxious mid-life women about their stressful situations. One 52-year-old woman, Moira, initially described herself as being 'on a roller-coaster of confusion', and her words are echoed by many of us when we cannot see 'the wood for the trees'. This happens when our lives are so crowded that we lose sight of our own selves.

Some women find that their brains are 'on the go' all the time, and when this occurs there is a clear knock-on effect from disturbed sleep patterns. Daily living is punctuated by erratic behaviour which disrupts normal physical, mental and spiritual functioning. If this strikes a chord with you, you need to know that you can help yourself. First, you need to create a quiet half an hour on your own every day with no interruptions so that you can

- identify where you are now
- reflect on and consider your options
- think about the elimination and/or better management of the stress in your life.

> " *I was 48 years old and had come to a crossroads in my life: I'd worked part-time as an estate agent to help my daughters through university and now wanted to do something different. I had being doing yoga for 20 years, and was encouraged to go on a teaching course in the Bahamas. It was very tough but I stuck with it and now teach three classes a week, as well as a class at the local golf club and private classes in people's homes. My dream is to have a health food restaurant with a yoga centre above it and alternative therapies on offer as well.*
>
> *I finally have a job that is more than merely a means to an end – I really enjoy the benefits I get from yoga and enjoy passing on those benefits to other people.*
>
> **JANET (London)** "

FROM CHAOS TO CLARITY

Step 1

You will need a large pad of paper and a pen. Divide one sheet of paper roughly into four sections and write the following words at the top of each one:

- Where am I now?
- Where do I want to be?
- How am I going to get there?
- What is stopping me?

Complete the sections with the words and thoughts that come immediately to mind – this should take about five or six minutes.

By focusing on the here-and-now, you put yourself, rather than the stressful situation, centre-stage. Maybe you have just drifted into your particular set of circumstances, with only a vague idea of what you were aiming for and putting your trust in fate. Now, your concentrated effort will bring secret hopes and desires to the surface, as well as allowing for the expression of unhappy feelings.

There may not yet be total clarity, but certain words and phrases may well be thought-provoking, so much so that you find yourself scribbling down other words and thoughts on another piece of paper. You have now begun the process of putting your particular 'roller-coaster' into some sort of perspective.

Step 2

The first step may have stirred up all manner of emotions for you, so this next one should be undertaken only when you feel ready for it. Read through everything you have written down and highlight stressful issues that need special attention.

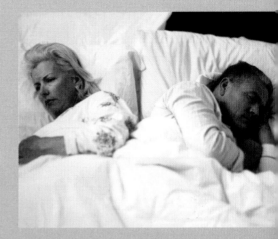

Sexual intimacy may be affected during the menopausal transition, and it will need patience and goodwill to re-establish.

Group them together under the following headings:

- My personal relationships
- My work outside my home

Select one of these and

- explore your options
- write down the possibilities for changes, even if some of them seem far-fetched
- formulate a plan of action.

If you are unsure about the best way forward, then a session with a counsellor may help you to resolve your uncertainties.

You could also benefit from incorporating one or more of the activities and therapies covered on pages 56–89 into your life. Start by learning to relax properly using the exercises on pages 72–73.

3

Natural alternatives

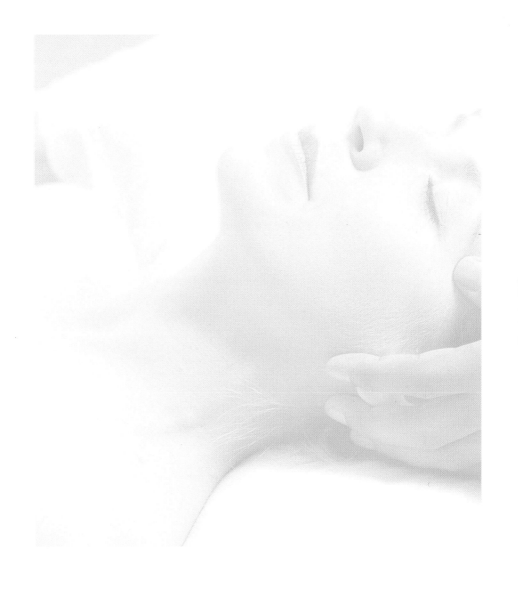

Considering the alternatives

Women are increasingly turning to natural remedies and complementary therapies to help alleviate menopausal symptoms. The main medical treatment for menopausal symptoms is hormone replacement therapy (HRT) and although this works well for some women, it can cause troublesome side-effects in others. You may even be told by your doctor that HRT is not appropriate for you because of your or your family's medical history – perhaps you have breast cancer in your family.

Or maybe you believe that any chemical interference in this transitional stage of your life is 'medicalizing' a normal event. Rather than treating your menopausal symptoms with drugs, you want to explore holistic alternatives.

Whatever your reason for choosing complementary therapies, you will find that there is a vast array of options to choose from. This chapter will give you an overview of the therapies that are most useful in treating menopausal symptoms. Some therapies, such as meditation, relaxation and yoga, are self-help techniques, while others, such as acupuncture and reflexology, require a consultation with a practitioner.

Natural alternatives

Every day, thousands of us seek help from acupuncturists, chiropractors, osteopaths, herbalists and homoeopaths, as well as practitioners of other therapies such as reflexology and aromatherapy. Why should there be such interest in complementary medicine, given the extraordinary achievements of orthodox medicine? It would be hard to exaggerate the benefits that have been obtained by applying scientific principles to medicine: most bacterial infections are curable, smallpox has been wiped out worldwide, and polio has ceased to be a major problem, at least in Western countries. Almost every week the media relays enthusiastic accounts of medical techniques or discoveries, such as organ transplantation; in-vitro fertilization and 'test-tube' babies; hip, knee and even arm replacements; cures for many cancers; and gene therapy.

And yet the fact is that much of this is divorced from the daily lives of most people. For women, it is frequently menstrual disorders that badly affect their lives, often presenting as depression, headaches, backache, water retention and premenstrual syndrome (PMS). The end result of an average six-minute interview with a harassed family doctor is most likely to be a prescription for antidepressants, painkillers, tranquillizers or sleeping tablets. Some of these are helpful in the short term, but many do not provide solutions and some even

Increasing the amount of exercise you do is a natural way to beat stress and anxiety and help you to feel more relaxed.

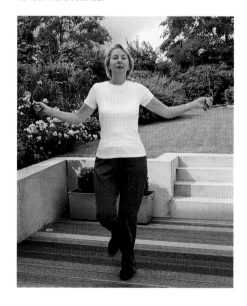

carry the potential risks of addiction and side-effects. In view of this, it is highly unlikely a therapy such as HRT could offer a universal panacea to women struggling through the 'change' from their reproductive to their post-reproductive years.

The fact that doctors are unable to guarantee the safety of prescribed drugs was all too clearly exemplified by the thalidomide tragedy in the late 1950s, when thousands of women who were given a drug to counteract morning sickness in pregnancy gave birth to children with severe limb deformities. Similarly, prescriptions of drugs such as Valium caused its users long-term problems. Medicine has also felt the winds of change as a climate of accountability has entered the arena. Many patients are much more medically literate than before, both as a direct result of medical trauma and because of the easy accessibility of information through the Internet. The suspicion of drugs and disenchantment with orthodox medicine has produced fertile ground for complementary medicine.

For years, the conventional medical community has been less than welcoming of complementary medicine – and with some justification. After all, in many places anyone could rent a room, buy a leather couch, put up a shiny brass plate on their door, preferably with a string of impressive-sounding letters after their name – and bingo! They were in business. They could be a real menace and danger to the potential patient. But how was the patient to know that?

The recognition of this problem eventually led many practitioners to put their houses in order: regulations, codes of ethics and competence, and validation now form benchmarks for public confidence and have paved the way for increasing collaboration with the conventional medical professions.

In the USA, a National Centre for

Complementary and Alternative Medicine (NCCAM) was set up in 1998 to explore these practices in the context of rigorous science, to train complementary and alternative researchers, and to disseminate the resulting information to the public and professionals. In March 2002 a White House Commission released a report promoting the wider use of complementary medicines. The report, which took nearly two years to complete, also called for more research into alternative therapies. The US budget for 2003 included over $100 million for this purpose. Unfortunately, however, researchers have yet to come up with evidence into treatment of menopausal symptoms by complementary medicine. This is perhaps surprising in view of the fact that a 1997 study conducted by the North American Menopause Society reported that 30 per cent of women use acupuncture, natural oestrogen(s), herbal supplements and phytoestrogens to relieve their symptoms.

Acupuncture

The use of acupuncture first caught the Western imagination around 1958 when it became recognized for its effectiveness in pain control, primarily for post-operative care. Later, it was introduced as an alternative to anaesthesia during operations, first with minor procedures such as tooth extraction and later with major operations performed on the limbs and abdomen.

Unfortunately, this dramatic use of acupuncture led to a widespread misconception about it, as its emphasis has

Fine, sterile needles are inserted into the skin at relevant points. They can be left in just briefly or inserted for about half-an-hour, depending on the condition.

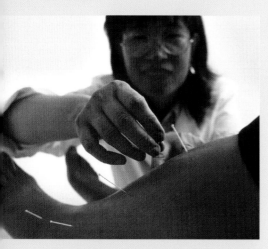

PAIN RELIEF

Legend has it that acupuncture was first discovered by a soldier shot by an arrow who found that, when struck by a second arrow, this relieved the pain from the first.

always been on prevention – to the Chinese, a sick man visiting an acupuncturist is comparable to a thirsty man starting to dig a well.

Acupuncture was first used widely in China and its history is closely connected with the development of Chinese medicine in general. The theory of Chinese medicine evolved out of an era of philosophical speculation and intense consideration of the nature of life by great thinkers such as Confucius. Its four methods of diagnosis – Observing, Listening and smelling, Asking, and Touching – remain as much the cornerstones of modern-day acupuncture treatment as they did in around 200BC, when a Chinese doctor, Bia Que, brought a prince out of a coma using acupuncture.

Central to the concept of acupuncture is the idea that the body is self-healing; that it is a self-rectifying whole, a network of interrelating and interacting energies. The even distribution and flow of these energies maintains health and any interruption, depletion or stagnation leads to disease. When this happens, acupuncture tries to aid the natural processes of healing, helping the body to correct itself by a realignment or redirection of energy which the Chinese call Qi (pronounced 'chee').

So what is Qi? It is often translated as breath, life-force or vitality – or simply as that which makes us alive. If there is no Qi, there is no life. Strong and energetic people have plenty of Qi; tired and depressed people lack Qi.

Along with the notion of Qi, acupuncture recognizes a subtle energy system by which Qi is circulated through the body in a network of channels or 'meridians'. The acupuncture points lie along these meridians and when the acupuncture needle is inserted, it is the Qi that is affected. In some ways, the circulation of Qi is similar to the blood circulation and nervous systems, although it is invisible to the eye.

Accepting this understanding of the body as an energetic and vibrating whole leads to a new approach to health and disease, for it draws together all the diverse signs and symptoms of ill-health to form a 'pattern of disharmony', which includes the mental/emotional state just as much as physical problems.

YIN AND YANG

The idea of harmony and balance forms the basis of the concept of 'yin' and 'yang'. The belief that each individual is governed by the opposing but complementary forces of yin and yang is central to all Chinese thought, because these forces are believed to affect everything in the universe.

Traditionally, yin is dark, passive, feminine, cold and negative, while yang is light, active, male, warm and positive. You and I might say that there are two opposing sides to everything, which are happy and sad, tired and energetic.

The Tai Chi symbol, shown above, illustrates how yin and yang flow into each other, with a little yin always within yang, and a little yang always within yin. The body, mind and emotions are all subject to these influences: when the two opposing forces are in balance we feel good, but if one force dominates the other, it brings about an imbalance which can result in ill-health. One of the main aims of the acupuncturist will be to restore and maintain your balance of yin and yang.

As you can see, acupuncture is not a system of medicine in isolation. It should be seen as one method of treatment within a complete system that has a different perspective on health from that of orthodox Western medicine. The idea of treating a patient's headaches in one medical department, their period pains in

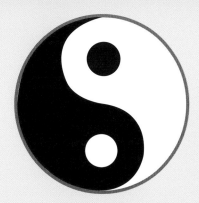

The Tai Chi symbol shows how yin and yang are opposites, but inseparable.

> " When I was 46, my periods suddenly became much heavier for six months with mid-cycle bleeding. The doctor diagnosed a fibroid and a hysterectomy was recommended. I was horrified and asked to see the acupuncturist – I am very fortunate, as complementary therapists work in the same premises as my family doctor, so all I had to do was walk down the corridor and make an appointment.
>
> The mid-cycle bleeding stopped after two treatments and my periods normalized for about 18 months. Then the mid-cycle bleeding started again and further treatment alleviated 90 per cent of this. By now I had realized I was menopausal, so continued with acupuncture for a further year during which time my periods stopped altogether.
>
> **CAROLINE (Somerset)** "

another and their insomnia in a third would seem extraordinary to an acupuncturist, since they believe there must be a common root.

Nowadays, a Westernized branch of acupuncture rejects the existence of channels or 'meridians' and believes that acupuncture

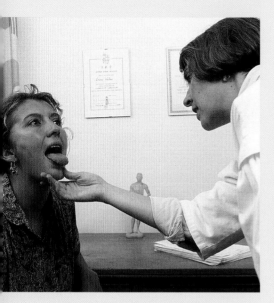

Your tongue can reveal a lot about the health of your organs.

PINPOINTING THE PROBLEM

During your first acupuncture consultation, time will be spent asking for details about your general condition. These questions can relate to all your physical, emotional and energetic signs and symptoms, and although some of them may seem unrelated, all can help the acupuncturist to form a more complete picture of your condition.

The practitioner will also ask to see your tongue. This tongue examination is a very important source of information for the acupuncturist: the shape, colour, coating and texture of the various parts of your tongue yield information about the state of your organs. A healthy tongue should be reddish in colour with little or no fur, it should not appear swollen or contracted, nor should there be cracks on the surface or 'teeth marks' along its sides.

During the consultation, a full medical history is taken. Other important questions concern:

- diet
- sleep patterns
- sensations of heat and cold, perspiration and whether this occurs during the day or night
- headaches – again, when they occur and in what part of the head
- urination and defecation, including frequency of passing urine and any tendency towards either constipation or diarrhoea.

works via the nervous system and that its effects can, in principle, be explained in terms of anatomy and physiology.

You will need to decide whether you are going to consult a lay practitioner (someone who may have had no formal training and possesses no accepted academic qualifications), or a doctor who is fully qualified through conventional medical training and who has undergone further training in acupuncture. Both types of practitioner are widely available.

WINNING APPROVAL

Acupuncture won the approval of the British Medical Association when a two-year study into its efficacy recommended in the year 2000 that it should be made more widely available to patients on the UK National Health Service.

If you consult an acupuncturist for treatment of menopausal problems, you will be asked about your menstrual cycle and the symptoms experienced. You will then be asked to undress, except for your underclothes, so that the acupuncturist can examine areas of your body that are painful, to feel for heat, cold, swelling, tightness or lack of skin tone. Specific acupuncture points may be touched to see if they are painful, particularly points on your abdomen and each side of your spine.

You may be surprised that the acupuncturist takes your pulse at both wrists and in three positions, by the index, middle and ring fingers. Acupuncturists believe that they can assess the balance of energy from these three positions and gain the key to your internal state. Your pulses will be checked again at intervals during treatment to monitor the energy changes.

Having gathered together all this information, the acupuncturist formulates the appropriate treatment for you. The choice of acupuncture points differs with each patient. Some points may be used repeatedly until a particular imbalance is corrected.

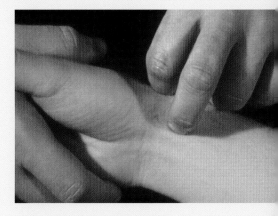

Taking accurate pulse readings on each wrist is a very important part of examination by an acupuncturist.

TREATMENT

Acupuncture stimulates the fine network of nerves running in the skin and sometimes nerves in the deeper tissues, too. These in turn affect the central nervous system, blocking pain and altering the nervous system's control of other bodily organs. Some patients show very little sensitivity to the needles and do not feel anything when they are inserted. Others may be aware of increased sensitivity in particular areas or on particular meridians. In general, however, treatment should not be painful and when needle sensation occurs it

should not last more than a few seconds. It is usually described as a 'tingling' sensation or a feeling of numbness radiating from the needle.

Treatment might be once a week to begin with, then at longer intervals as the condition responds – it depends on you and your 'pattern of disharmony'. It is demonstrably untrue to say that the results of acupuncture are 'all in the mind'. After all, treatments have been successfully carried out on very small children and animals. It is very unlikely that a cow could be hypnotized into improved health by a veterinary surgeon!

SAFETY FIRST

Before undergoing any treatment, you should ask about the sterilization procedures in use at the clinic. In the UK and many other countries all registered acupuncturists are required by law to sterilize needles. Disposable needles are available if you prefer, though they will obviously be more expensive.

DID YOU KNOW?

The symptoms of just over 50 per cent of 300 menopausal women disappeared when treated with acupuncture at the First Hospital, Tianjin, China in 1998.

Traditional Chinese medicine

Traditional Chinese medicine incorporates not only acupuncture but also herbal medicines, dietary suggestions, massage and/or exercises or lifestyle recommendations. It would appear that Chinese medicinal herbs are more effective when they are used in conjunction with the other elements of traditional Chinese medicine.

Because of its holistic view of the body and mind, a course of Chinese medicine will be designed in response to each patient's individual needs. For example, five different women coming into a clinic complaining of hot flushes will have a variety of different accompanying signs and symptoms, no two of which are exactly alike. Therefore, each woman will receive an individually tailored treatment plan with different herbs, different acupuncture therapies and different suggestions for lifestyle changes.

According to traditional Chinese medicine, the clinical picture of hot flushes shows a deterioration in the yin of the Liver, weakness in the Blood of the Heart, and an exhaustion of the Water of the Kidney.

The deficiency of Water is countered by an excess of Fire, which endangers the control of the yin of the Liver and unleashes its yang. There are two pathological mechanisms:

- The combined effects of deficiency in the Kidney, hyperactivity in the Liver and flare-up of Heart Fire will lead to palpitations, insomnia and dizziness.
- The imbalance between the Spleen and Liver is manifested by emotional depression, irritability, loss of temper and an oppressive feeling in the chest.

Medicinal herbs are just one part of traditional Chinese medicine.

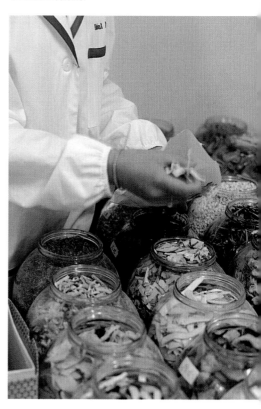

CONTRADICTORY EVIDENCE

Chinese herbal medicine has been used for centuries in China for treating menopausal symptoms, and some clinical trials there have shown it to be very effective.

However, a placebo-controlled trial using Chinese medicinal herbs to treat 55 menopausal women in Australia (1998–1999) found they were no more effective than placebo in reducing hot flushes and night sweats.

TAI CHI

T'ai chi chuan, also known as Tai Chi, is a fitness regimen that was developed specifically to promote the flow of Qi (life-force energy) within the body.

Through slow, flowing movements, Tai Chi increases your strength and muscle tone, enhances your range of motion and flexibility, and improves your balance and coordination. Practitioners of traditional Chinese medicine believe that although the movements of Tai Chi are low impact and low intensity, they have the power to break up blockages of Qi in the body and re-establish the flow of this vital force.

All Tai Chi movements are pairs of opposites: for example, left and right, and yield and thrust. This reflects the attempt to harmonize the two opposing forces of yin and yang (see page 59).

Tai Chi is a form of moving meditation in which precise movements and controlled breathing are synchronized to enable the practitioner to flow with the direction of energy in and around the body. Its movements of stepping, shifting weight and rotating have been compared to yoga and ballet.

The beneficial effects of Tai Chi are similar to those of Western aerobic exercise, but without the stresses and strains. Tai Chi has been practised for centuries in China. Now, people all over the world practise this ancient discipline in parks, community centres and health clubs.

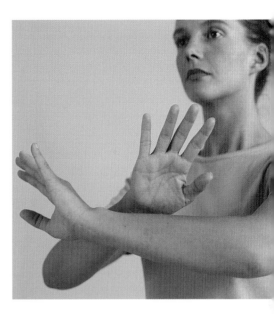

The harmonious movements of Tai Chi can have a positive effect on your physical and psychological well-being.

How Tai Chi can help during the menopause

Tai Chi offers a variety of physical and psychological benefits, such as improved cognitive function and decreased levels of anxiety, depression, stress and muscular tension, as well as improved circulation and enhanced energy and well-being.

DID YOU KNOW?
Legend has it that the movements of Tai Chi are based on those of a snake. The story goes that a martial arts master was inspired by the mutual movements of a snake and a crane in a lethal dance of attack and evasion. The graceful and controlled way the snake dodged and counter-attacked became the basis for the movement of Tai Chi.

Medical herbalism

There can be little doubt that plants were the first source of medicines, and the use of herbs as a source of healing remedies is inherent in all cultures in all historical times. Today, using herbs to nurture and heal the body is a thriving complementary therapy. You can buy herbal remedies in health food shops and pharmacies or via a website. Alternatively, you can consult a fully qualified medical herbalist.

In every rural community since pre-history there have been individuals who have been regarded as specialists in the art of using healing plants. Their knowledge has been passed down from one generation to the next, resulting in the creation of an enormous body of information about the medicinal value of plants. Although herbal practices were pushed into relative obscurity during the nineteenth and twentieth centuries, there was a renewed interest in medical herbalism at the end of the last century. People who feel uneasy about the widespread use of drugs and their side-effects often welcome the natural and holistic aspects of herbalism.

Many different herbs are used to make up the complex herbal preparations that are the mainstay of medical herbalism.

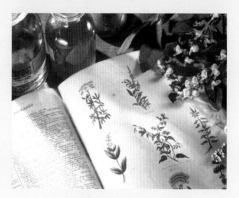

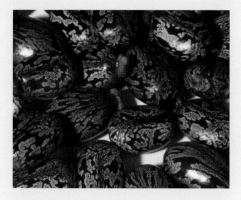

The beans of the castor tree have been used for their purgative properties for hundreds of years.

66 *I consulted a private doctor last autumn, desperate for a way to overcome hot flushes, and her remedies have been astonishingly successful. I take Menosan drops, a tincture made from the herb sage, three times every day plus one red clover tablet once daily. Supplements and a cream have eased a few other problems that have begun or have become worse in the past two to three years.*

LINDA (London) 99

THE CONSULTATION
The herbalist will give you a thorough examination and will take details of your medical history and eating lifestyle. Your blood pressure will be checked and the practitioner will evaluate the overall balance of your body's systems – musculo-skeletal, nervous, cardiovascular, digestive, genito-urinary and endocrine – to discover underlying and predisposing disharmonies.

It is you as a whole person who will be treated, not simply the complaint. Thus, entirely different remedies may be prescribed

HERBS COMMONLY USED FOR PERI-MENOPAUSAL AND MENOPAUSAL SYMPTOMS

Name of herb	For relief of	Recommendations
Balm	Tension, stress reactions and depression	A tincture of 2-6 ml 3 times a day, or 2-3 teaspoons of dried herb steeped in 1 cup of boiling water twice a day
Black cohosh	Hot flushes, anxiety and depression	40–200 mg daily - use not to exceed six months
Chastetree berry	Hot flushes	Prepared as a tincture, chastetree berry provides an average daily dose equal to 20 mg of the crude fruit or 30-40 mg of the fruit in a decoction
Gingko	Poor memory, mood swings, anxiety and absent-mindedness	A daily dose of 120-160 mg of standardized gingko leaf extract
Ginseng	Fatigue, diminished work capacity and loss of concentration	500 mg capsule can be taken 3-6 times a day – use not to exceed three months
St John's wort	Depression	2-4 g of hypericin capsule 1-2 times a day. The equivalent may be steeped in 1 cup of boiling water for 10 minutes to gain a similar amount
Valerian	Insomnia and tension	2-3 g, taken 1-3 times a day, is suggested as an anti-anxiety regimen

to two patients apparently suffering from the same problems.

You are unlikely to need frequent consultations unless you have a condition that requires close monitoring and regular examinations. You can simply telephone the herbalist when you need more medicine and any adjustments can be made to the remedy if necessary.

Many patients note a measurable degree of improvement within the first month of treatment, but one to two months of treatment for every year of illness may be required if the condition is chronic.

SAFETY

It is a persistent and popular misconception that herbal medicines are totally safe and free from side-effects. However, this is far from true – after all, many plants from which the remedies are made are known to be poisonous. Under the terms of the UK Medicines Act 1968, herbal practitioners are permitted to use a few poisonous plants, such as aconite, belladonna, mandrake, hemlock and white bryony, up to statutory maximum dosages, but these are not permitted for general sale. Similar regulations apply in other countries.

FORMS OF HERBAL PREPARATION

Preparation	Description
Bulk herbs	Raw, dried plant material in jars or bins; used in teas, tinctures; powdered for capsules, tablets
Oils	External use only, some are fatal if ingested; used in aromatherapy
Tablets, capsules	Stored and transported easily
Teas	Hot-water extracts, of which there are three types: Beverages, teas - steeped for 1-2 minutes Infusions - steeped for 10-20 minutes Decoctions - plant material simmered in boiling water for 10-20 minutes
Tinctures	Alcohol extracts; highly concentrated; come in small bottles with eyedropper caps; few drops usually used

In 1978 Germany established Commission E to review the safety and use of over 1,400 herbal drugs. The seven herbs in the table on page 65 were considered by Commission E to be effective and safe for one or more peri-menopausal or menopausal complaints.

In Germany alone, 10 million prescriptions for gingko are written each year by more than 10,000 physicians.

HERBAL PREPARATIONS

Herbal medicines come in various forms, some of which are ready for use and some of which require preparation.

Many people choose to buy ready-made preparations, but others prefer to buy the raw materials and create their own remedies. Breaking down the herb samples to a suitable size used to be the hardest part of preparation,

SAFETY CONCERNS

Much of the concern about the safety, efficacy and quality of herbal remedies may be removed following the European Union's traditional herbal medicines directive, which came into force at the end of 2002. This will require manufacturers to register unlicensed products and produce them according to good pharmaceutical manufacturing practice.

BLACK COHOSH

At present, the most effective herbal medicine for treating menopausal symptoms is an extract of black cohosh, Remifemin (known as RemiFemin in the USA), which has been subjected to two clinical trials. The safety profile is positive with low toxicity, few and mild side-effects and good tolerability. Remifemin has been used in Germany since the 1950s.

entailing hours of labour with a pestle and mortar, but nowadays a kitchen blender will perform many functions quite adequately.

Water or a mixture of water and ethyl alcohol is usually added to the herbs. Sometimes acetic acid (vinegar), glycerol (or glycerine) and seed oils are used. A liquid is selected that will have the best chance of dissolving the required active ingredients. 'Woody' material such as bark and roots has to be infused in hot water for a certain period.

Being natural products, herbal preparations are very variable in strength. The quantity of active ingredients will differ widely from product to product. The raw material will vary according to the climate and conditions in which it is grown, and the quality of the preparation will vary according to how it is treated and how many other ingredients are added. In addition, the dosage will depend on how you prepare it – for example, the longer teas are steeped, the stronger the dose.

COMBINING MEDICINES

Your medical herbalist will not advise you to stop taking drugs prescribed by your doctor and will usually work together with any orthodox treatment deemed necessary. Many patients want to come off their prescribed drugs and herbalists would aim to reduce or eliminate the need for them.

SENSIBLE MEASURES

In general, herbal medicines may have a short-term role in managing the symptoms of menopause, but they are unlikely to be useful in treating the long-term aspects, in particular osteoporosis. Never persist with any herbal remedy if, after a period of no more than several weeks, it is not clearly improving your condition. Most herbs do not take months to work. Always challenge a treatment if you do not think it is useful.

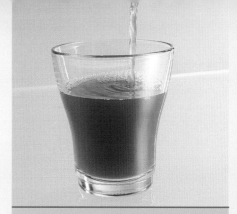

INFUSIONS

To make an infusion, use 1 teaspoon of dried herbs to 1 cup of boiling water; leave to infuse for 10-15 minutes, strain and drink hot. Sweeten with honey if preferred.

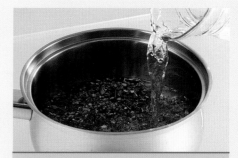

DECOCTIONS

These are made from materials such as roots, barks, nuts and seeds. Using the same proportion as for an infusion, place the mixture and water in a saucepan. Bring to the boil, then simmer for 10 minutes. Strain and drink hot.

Homoeopathy

Nearly two hundred years ago, an eminent and conventionally qualified German physician published the first results of a form of treatment which he had developed and used experimentally on himself and his family. His name was Samuel Hahnemann and he christened the principle of this treatment 'homoeopathy', from two Greek words – *homios* meaning 'like' and *pathos* meaning 'suffering'.

In some ways Hahnemann was a scientist, but in others he was a metaphysician or even a mystic. He believed that life was sustained by a vital force and that disease was caused by some outside influence that disturbed the smooth functioning of the vital force, thus inducing symptoms of illness. His belief was that if you could discover and remove the cause of the trouble and stimulate the vital healing force of nature, then the patient would heal themselves.

It had all begun when Hahnemann decided to see what would happen if he dosed himself with quinine, a remedy used to combat malaria. He was surprised to find that he developed a fever and other symptoms associated with malaria, even though he did not have the disease. These symptoms then disappeared when he stopped taking it. But each time he dosed himself again with quinine, the symptoms recurred. Here was confirmation of Hippocrates' belief that if an individual who is suffering from an illness can be made to suffer symptoms similar to those produced by his illness, then he will be cured, and that the severity of symptoms and healing responses are dependent on the individual.

This 'like cures like' principle formed the basis of homoeopathy and is in stark contrast to conventional or 'allopathic' medicine, which treats illness with an antidote rather than a similar substance. But this was not the only

Onions are just one of the substances that are used for homoeopathic remedies.

Sage can be taken to help reduce hot flushes.

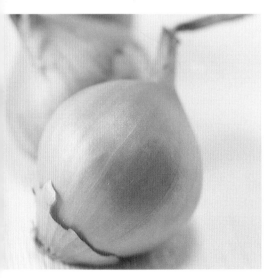

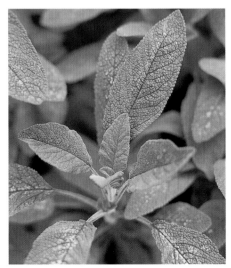

PUT TO THE TEST

A total of 657 patients received homoeopathic treatment for their pre- and post-menopausal complaints in a three-month study conducted in 1994 by 77 therapists in Germany.

Participants were given Mulimen, a combination homoeopathic preparation consisting of agnus castus, black cohosh, ambergris, St John's wort, common nettle, sepia, calcium, potassium and gelsenium.

Two-thirds reported continuous and definite relief from their symptoms, and even though they did not achieve complete freedom from them, all stated their intention to continue with Mulimen.

principle that distinguished Hahnemann's medical practice from that of his contemporaries. Dissatisfied with the medical practices of his day, which consisted mainly of 'bleeding' and the use of large doses of dangerous drugs, he decided to dispense smaller doses of medicine. To his surprise, he found that the more the remedy was diluted, the more active it became.

Orthodox medicine was unimpressed. This paradox – that less of a substance could be more effective – was perhaps not surprisingly unacceptable to the scientific community of the time, as well as to modern sceptics who doubt the worth of giving extremely dilute solutions of dubious substances to the sick. Nevertheless, every year 4 per cent of adults in the USA use a homoeopathic medicine, while in the UK the figure is more than double that at 8.5 per cent.

Hahnemann and his followers were ridiculed, yet they continued to experiment with all sorts of substances – derived from minerals or animal and plant products – testing them in what he termed 'provings'. Over long periods they took small doses of various reputedly poisonous or medicinal substances, carefully noting the symptoms produced. Patients who were suffering from similar symptoms were then treated with these substances, with encouraging results.

An enormous amount of information was accumulated to form the main source of knowledge about homoeopathy. By the time he died in 1843, Hahnemann had done 'provings' on 99 substances. This increased to 600 more medicines by 1900 and today there are nearly 3,000 substances available to homoeopaths. The materials include onion, Indian hemp, honey-bee sting venom, snake venom and spiders, as well as sand, charcoal, common salt and pencil lead. Hahnemann also advocated the use of single medicines rather than complex mixtures, reasoning that it was not possible to distinguish the effects of large numbers of drugs when they were all mixed together.

There are two forms of homoeopathy in use today: one which lays great emphasis on the use of highly dilute medicines and on certain philosophical, even semi-mystical ideas about disease and its causation, and a modern form that is based on fairly orthodox notions of pharmacology and largely ignores philosophical thought. But the essence of the homoeopathic principle remains the same: it is the patient who is treated rather than the disease.

• Graphites for irritability, difficulty in concentrating, depression, weepiness and over-excitability

However, it can be difficult to evaluate your own situation clearly, and consulting a homoeopath for a professional opinion will result in the correctly chosen remedy in the right potency. The homoeopath might be a lay practitioner (someone who may have had no formal training and possesses no accepted academic qualifications) or a doctor who is fully qualified through conventional medical training and who has undergone further training in homoeopathy.

THE CONSULTATION

Your first homoeopathy appointment may last as long as two hours, as making the correct diagnosis is a vitally important part of the treatment. A lot will need to be known about you in order to build up a multi-dimensional picture of you as an individual:

Sage can be taken as an infusion, tincture, ointment, massage rub, compress or mouthwash.

HOMOEOPATHIC REMEDIES

A single remedy may be prescribed from a variety of sources and in a number of dilutions, such as Pulsatilla (an anemone flower), Sepia (a sea creature) or Sulphur (a mineral). The homoeopath has thousands of remedies to choose from and the process of selecting the right one is a carefully considered one. However, there are several remedies that are readily available in pharmacies and health food shops, such as:

• Lachesis for poor memory, difficulty in concentrating, anxiety and depression
• Pulsatilla for depression, weepiness, changeable moods and headaches
• Argentum nitricum (Arg. nit.) and Salvia (sage) for hot flushes

• Your past health and life circumstances, the pattern of health in your family, your present condition.
• What are the particular symptoms? What makes them worse or better – warmth, cold, eating, drinking, moving about, lying down and so on?
• How do you feel about the condition (angry, resentful, depressed)?
• What are your underlying fears, moods and anxieties?

Having gathered all the information needed, and assuming that you do not need to be referred to a doctor, then the homoeopath will analyse the answers you have supplied and formulate the appropriate medicine. This can then be obtained from your pharmacist.

Although they are completely different in their preparation and action, homoeopathic medicines look much like any other medicine, and are taken in the form of small pills, tablets, drops, granules, powders and liquids.

SAFETY

Homoeopathic remedies are completely safe, non-toxic and non-addictive.

COMBINING MEDICINES

It is perfectly safe to take antibiotics along with a homoeopathic medicine, though the side-effects from the antibiotic may complicate the symptoms picture and thus make the choice of homoeopathic treatment more difficult.

A number of homoeopathic substances have a very specific application in certain conditions, such as indigestion and bruising, and so they can successfully treat a large cross-section of

Pulsatilla is recommended to treat depression, insomnia and conditions of the reproductive system.

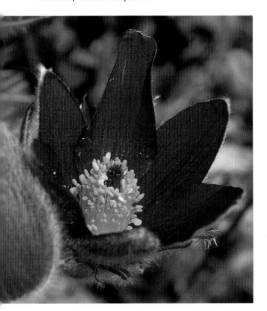

the population. For instance, arnica ointment is very effective for healing bruises following an operation.

Some feeling of well-being is usually experienced within one week, even though the symptoms remain. However, if symptoms do not improve within two weeks of starting treatment, then an alternative medicine should be considered.

"

I consulted a registered homoeopath, who spent one-and-a-half hours asking me a number of questions about my general health, my current situation, major events in my life, and seemingly unrelated questions such as 'How do you feel about frogs? and thunderstorms?' She reassured me that my symptoms of irritability, mood swings, change in sexual desire, irregular and heavy bleeding, random sweating, weight gain, sleeplessness and palpitations were common when women were peri-menopausal. Having listened carefully, she then prescribed a remedy for me - pulsatilla.

The first week I took it, I experienced violent mood swings and severe irritability to the point where I almost felt out of control. I had decided to give it one more week and then give up if there was no improvement and, as if by magic, everything changed. I slept better, my periods became more regular and the bleeding lessened, my mood evened out and I became altogether much more pleasant to be with, both for my family and myself.

I would not hesitate to recommend homoeopathy for this stage of a woman's life.

VICKI (Bristol)

"

Learning to relax

You may think – oh, that's easy! I relax every time I come home from work, kick off my shoes and flop into a comfortable chair with my favourite tipple. And yes, some of your tension will fall away, as you relax initially in a passive, unfocused way. But not all of it will disappear, for most of us have been conditioned to believe that we must constantly be active and productive, so our minds are likely to be preoccupied with all sorts of issues that we feel are important.

Many of us assume that relaxation comes naturally to us, but in fact it does not. Setting aside time to carry out the two exercises detailed opposite is a simple way to start

practising *really* letting go. It may well feel a bit strange at first, but the effect of deep relaxation can be both releasing and rejuvenating. These exercises can be practised while you are lying in bed before falling asleep, or at any time when you want to achieve really deep relaxation. They feature three distinctive elements:

- Focusing on particular muscles
- Tension in holding them
- Relaxation

When you relax properly your entire body will be loose and totally at ease.

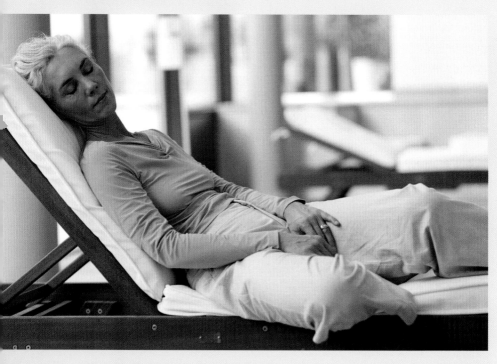

EXERCISE 1: A Breathing Space

Your surroundings need to be warm and comfortable, and your clothes loose-fitting. If you try this exercise on the floor, place an additional covering over it such as a large piece of foam rubber, a futon or duvet.

1   Get into your chosen position and close your eyes.
2   Focus on your breathing – feel how the air goes in and out of your lungs.
3   Feel the weight and warmth of your body – as you relax deeper into yourself, you will feel even heavier as the warmth begins to envelop you.
4   Take a deep breath, expanding your diaphragm and ribs, hold it for two seconds, then sigh, releasing all the air from your lungs. Listen to the air as it is expelled. Repeat this 5–6 times.

From shoulder to shoulder

Hold each position to an even count of 5.

5   Hunch your shoulders as high as you can – hold them there – relax.
6   Tense the upper part of your arms – hold – relax.
7   Tense your complete arms – hold – relax.
8   Clench your fists – hold – relax.

On a lower level

9   Tense your buttocks – hold – relax. Do the same with your thighs and the calf muscles in your legs.
10 Draw your feet up in the direction of your upper body, as if you are straining to see them – hold – relax.
11 Curl your toes – hold – relax.

You are now fully relaxed, and may drift off to sleep – or you can return gradually to consciousness by counting down from 10 to 1.

EXERCISE 2: Relaxation and Mental Imagery

Mental imagery, also known as visualization, means forming an image in your mind, then creating a clear mental statement of what you want to happen.

Some of us are more 'visual' than others. Some people think primarily in images, whereas others tend to sense or feel things, and some people think in words. You need to operate in the sense that is most natural to you in visualizing your desired outcome.

For example, if you have high blood pressure, you could visualize the problem as little muscles in the walls of your blood vessels tightening down, so that it causes much higher pressure than is necessary for the blood to be driven through. Now, see the medication relaxing the muscles in the blood vessels, your heart pumping with less resistance, and blood flowing through the vascular channels.

1   Set yourself a mental goal: for instance, the relief of repeated anxious feelings.
2   Prepare yourself with the relaxation exercises (see left).
3   Retreat in your mind to a special place, perhaps a tropical beach. Allow yourself to use all your senses to explore it – to feel the warm sun, smell the plants, listen to the birds, feel the salt spray on your body, the sand tickling your toes.
4   When your special place is established, put yourself into the image to achieve your goal – a relaxed mind is receptive to anything you want to give it.
5   Make a positive mental statement about yourself – 'I feel calm and in control'.
6   Drift away gradually from your special place. When you open your eyes, you will feel relaxed and refreshed. Do not get up immediately, as the drop in blood pressure may make you feel giddy.

Meditation

Meditation aims to achieve both relaxation of the body and a heightened state of awareness. Regular meditation can bring greater control over restless thoughts and emotions, leading to a sense of well-being, and as a result you will be able to shut yourself off from the world and find inner peace.

It is now generally accepted that our minds can influence mechanical bodily functions and the chemical balance that ensures good health. When our minds are persistently disturbed by unhappy thoughts and feelings, such as worry, anxiety and resentment, then our energy levels become disrupted, and these then manifest as physical symptoms of illness.

Meditation can offer considerable benefits. It has been found to be effective in:

- regulating blood pressure
- stimulating blood circulation
- alleviating pain
- reducing muscular tension
- slowing down hormonal activity.

Although meditation is often associated with an ascetic, spiritual lifestyle, there is no need for you to renounce your own beliefs. It is enough for you to approach your meditation practice as just another element in your daily exercise routine, and take from it whatever you feel you need – be it relief from stress, improved physical and mental health, or a sustained sense of well-being.

When you first start meditating, it is important to try to establish good habits, specifically those concerning correct posture and breath control. Both of these are useful in aiding your concentration when your thoughts wander, as inevitably they will in the early stages of meditation.

POSTURE

Although the various postures described on these pages are interchangeable, you could attempt all of them initially, persevering with each for a week until settling with one or two that suit you.

Lying down

If you choose to lie down on your back, make sure you support your neck with a cushion. Let your arms hang loosely by your side and keep your legs straight. Do not cross your legs or put your hands on your body.

This is a comfortable position to relax in. Simply kneel on the floor, place a cushion behind your knees and sit down.

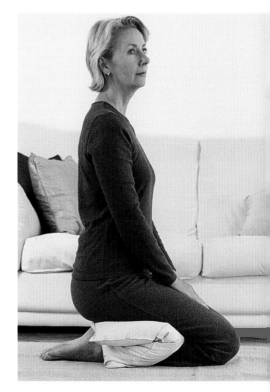

Sitting

Choose a straight-backed chair to sit in so that you are supported and do not cramp your diaphragm. Your feet should be flat on the floor and slightly apart, in line with your shoulders. Place your hands on your knees, palms down, although you may prefer to have them facing upwards in a symbolic gesture of openness.

Classical postures

The traditional cross-legged postures that are used in yoga require a degree of suppleness you may not possess. An alternative to the classical postures is to rest on your heels with a cushion supporting your buttocks, as in the Japanese tradition.

STARTING TO MEDITATE

Without doubt, when you first learn to meditate the most difficult aspect is the quietening of the mind. Initially, you will probably find lots of other things that seem in more urgent need of your attention and you will be tempted to put off your meditation time indefinitely.

It is important to begin with simple exercises to establish good practice. This basic candle gazing meditation will help you to establish the habit of sitting still in silence and will train your mind to focus on the object of the exercise. Practise it twice a day for six days, then rest for one day before moving on to the other meditations described on pages 76–77.

Candle gazing

1   Place a candle in front of you, so that the candle is in line with the point between your eyebrows.
2   Gaze at the candle and observe the flicker, size and every aspect of it.
3   After 30–60 seconds, close your eyes, and keep the flame as steady as you can. At first the afterglow will fade and you will be left with nothing, so you will need to open your

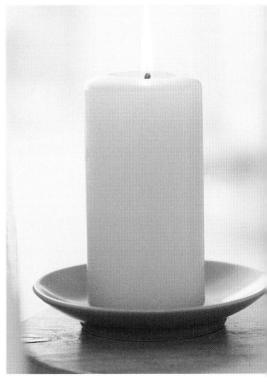

Learn to meditate by training your mind to focus on the flickering flame of a candle.

eyes again, and repeat the process. You will then retain an optical image of the candle and the flicker of light in your mind.
4   When the flicker of light starts to disappear, force the image to stay. This trains your mind to concentrate hard. At first it will seem impossible to maintain the image, but with continued practice it becomes easy.
5   Focus your attention on one thought, and keep breathing deeply while still focusing your mind on it.
6   Become one with the flame so that there is no space between it and you. Enjoy the sense of spaciousness and expansion.
7   When you feel ready, slowly come back to waking consciousness and open your eyes.

OTHER MEDITATIONS

Helpful meditations in your present circumstances could include the following.

Pain reduction – the ball

1   Prepare yourself with the relaxation exercises on pages 72–73.
2   Focus on your pain. What colour is it? See its colour, shape and size clearly. It may be a red ball. It may be the size of a tennis ball or a grapefruit.
3   Mentally project the ball out into space, maybe two metres away from your body.
4   Make the ball bigger, about the size of a football, then shrink it to the size of a pea. Now let it become whatever size it chooses to be.

Writing a letter may help you to release your anger.

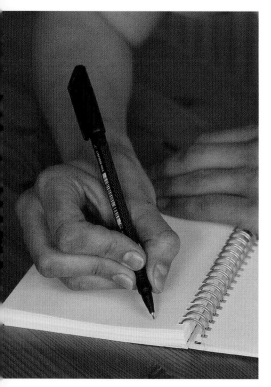

5   Begin to change the ball's colour – make it pink, then light green.
6   Now take the green ball and put it back where you originally saw it. At this point, notice whether or not your pain has been reduced.

Pain reduction – the blanket

1   Prepare yourself with the relaxation exercises on pages 72–73.
2   When you feel relaxed, imagine that a thick, full-length blanket is being wrapped around your being. Enjoy the relief it brings and the sense of heat that envelops your body.
3   Let the heat penetrate into the very core of you so that any pain or discomfort starts to fade. Allow yourself to feel a sensation of detachment.
4   Visualize your pain as something physical, such as smoke or grit, that is being drawn out of your body to be absorbed by the blanket, leaving your body cleansed.
5   When you feel that the last bit of smoke or grit has left you, imagine throwing off the blanket and watching it disintegrate, taking your pain along with it.
6   End the meditation by visualizing a ball of dazzling bright light over your head. Watch it as it slowly moves down towards your feet and and dissolves into the floor. Return to normal and observe the effect of the meditation on your pain.

Getting rid of an upset

1   Take up your chosen relaxed position.
2   Close your eyes, breathe naturally, and when you feel suitably relaxed, imagine that you are sitting at a desk. In front of you are pen, paper, envelope, candle, matches and a bowl filled with water.
3   Look down at the blank paper in front of you and take up the pen.
4   Now write a letter to the person whom you

believe has upset you, describing your feelings and explaining the situation as you understand it. It is necessary to express your feelings, as the primary purpose of this exercise is to face and free your emotions. Once you have released your anger, you will hopefully see the situation from a less impassioned perspective, and having done so, you may well feel in a position to 'forgive and forget'.

5   When you have finished writing your letter, imagine addressing the envelope and put the letter inside.

6   Visualize lighting the candle. Hold the envelope over the flame, and when it has curled into ashes, drop it into the bowl.

7   When you feel ready, slowly come back to waking consciousness and open your eyes.

Relationship problems

It takes two to create difficulties in any relationship, and it can be very hard to break the 'blaming' habit.

1   Take up your chosen relaxed position.

2   Close your eyes, breathe naturally, and when you feel suitably relaxed, visualize the other person.

3   Soften your heart centre by meditating on compassion.

4   See the other person as a being whose human nature is as fallible as your own.

5   Draw them towards you and embrace them, while repeating the following affirmation: 'You and I are enjoying a good, positive relationship. Energy is flowing freely between us'. Then release them and watch as they fade into the distance.

Tension will be diffused and you will be able to talk through matters calmly.

Getting a grip on fear

This meditation can be done prior to and even during a situation or activity that is causing you anxiety. You will be surprised at how much better you feel.

1   The simplest method of dispelling immediate anxiety is also the most effective. Simply take the deepest breath that you can, and hold it for a moment before exhaling. The result is instantaneous. It not only restores your heartbeat to its regular rhythm and reduces the flow of adrenalin, but it also allows a pause in which you can reassume control, calm your mind and clarify your thoughts.

2   Repeat the first step but, as you inhale, imagine that you are drawing up fear or anxiety in the form of stale air or smoke from deep within your body. As you exhale, imagine that all your fear and anxiety is flowing out of you.

3   Now add this visualization to the previous step: close your eyes, relax and take a long, deep breath. When you exhale, imagine that you are blowing up a balloon. Pause, then take another breath. Each time you exhale, imagine that you are filling the balloon with fear and anxiety. When the balloon is stretched to bursting, mentally tie the knot and seal your fear inside. Now take great pleasure in popping the balloon and dispersing all your negative feelings.

Getting away from it all

Many women in their menopausal years feel as though they are swept along by a tide of events beyond their control, without a chance for a little peaceful living. Our lives are filled with preoccupations, distractions and responsibilities, and however much we may yearn for peace, there seems little chance of making the time and space for it.

Going on retreat is a deliberate attempt to step outside ordinary life; to create a place and time of peace and quiet where distractions are at a minimum. Here is a space for you to contemplate the deepest feelings and thoughts about yourself and your relationships. Everything we feel and do is filtered through our sense of self – call it self-awareness, self-identity or consciousness, it is intrinsic to being a human.

In doing so, you may find a surprising void – an empty inner space you never knew existed. Suddenly there are no friends, children, partners, pets, television, work or the constant background of human activity. There is no gossip, no grumbling, no meetings, no decisions, no interference – you are faced with you alone. You begin to slip into a slower physical, mental and emotional gear and start to think differently – taking stock is what going on retreat is all about.

WHO GOES ON RETREAT?

People of all ages and from all walks of life take advantage of the benefits of going on retreat – students, homemakers, grandparents, businessmen and women, millionaire celebrities and the unknown poor. Men and women of all faiths and those of none go on retreat.

You will find many different types of retreat advertised in magazines and on the internet. Most aim towards self-discovery of an experiential nature, and they can vary in duration from just a single day to a week or more.

Day retreats These can be very flexible. It might be a day for silence, a day based on a theme or an activity-centred day, a time for group discussion or talks, or for lessons given in meditation technique.

Weekend retreats These are often run along the following lines: you arrive on Friday evening, and, after settling your things in your room, meet the retreat leader and other guests. After supper you meet for a short talk about the weekend and are given a timetable. From that time onwards you will cease talking unless it is to the retreat leader, or during a group discussion or shared prayer. There will be time for walks, reading and just resting – simple, easy and peaceful.

Going on retreat means that you will have lots of time for reading, resting and quiet contemplation.

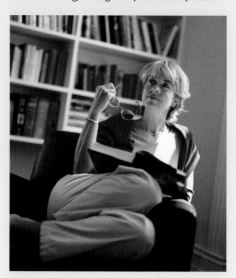

Healing retreats These may use prayer, meditation, chanting or the laying-on of hands. Healing may be concerned with a physical complaint or with healing the whole person in order to eliminate obstacles to personal and spiritual growth.

Lesbian retreats These often have themes that bear directly on living as a lesbian within society and which link into spiritual matters.

Private retreats In these you go alone as an individual. It is usually a silent time in which you find solitude in order to reflect, rest and meditate. In many monasteries and retreat houses, you may arrange to take your meals in your room or separately from others so that you can maintain this framework of silence.

Embroidery, calligraphy and painting retreats Themed retreats focus on awakening personal creativity through a craft or art form. There are many other subjects as themes, such as pottery, poetry, music or gardening.

Having placed yourself among strangers, you may meet people you like at once, those you do not want to know better, as well as those who make a nuisance of themselves – the sort of person who has some problem and cannot help talking about it. Equally, you may encounter those who are certain their beliefs hold the key to life. If you do not want to listen to them, then walk away – alternatively, you might find it both charitable and instructive to really listen to what the person is saying, even if you do not believe a word of it. And you do not have to discuss any of your beliefs or feelings unless you want to do so.

Going on retreat is about refreshing yourself, relaxing and taking a journey into your deeper self. Reassessment of your life and relationships and values can happen. And why not? When have you ever had time to do this?

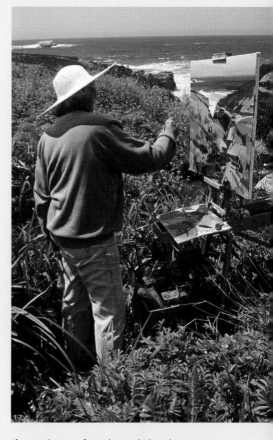

If you enjoy a craft, such as painting, then a retreat that allows you to focus on your creativity might suit you.

BEFORE YOU BOOK...
If you have a disability, you will need to double-check the facilities before booking, as many retreat centres and their guest accommodation have not yet been updated to the national standard set for the disabled.

Yoga

Yoga is often seen as a mystical Eastern relaxation system, which involves intricate postures that only the most supple and double-jointed of us would dare to attempt. But as many people have discovered, the movements can be very simple and beneficial whether you are 9 or 90 years old, even if your joints are creaking or you are ill or disabled.

Its original practitioners some 4,000 years ago in ancient India were philosophers or yogis who lived as hermits. Today, the benefits of yoga have spread internationally and it is now practised in non-religious, non-cultural-based classes all over the Western world, from local adult education classes in village halls to centres and organizations devoted exclusively to yoga. This ancient way to better health has been adopted by people of all ages and from all walks of life.

Most classes are based on hatha yoga or physical yoga – *ha* means the sun, which represents masculine energy, and *tha* means the moon, representing feminine energy.

BASIC UNDERSTANDINGS

The three principles of hatha yoga are:

- **Pranayama (breathing)** This breathing technique encourages us to make full use of our lungs, balances the masculine and feminine energies within our bodies, and boosts energy levels.
- **Asanas (postures)** These are held for as long as possible, in order to build stamina as well alter the energy in our bodies.
- **Dhyana (meditation)**.

Stretching is the best way to achieve top-to-toe fitness as well as reducing stress in your groups of muscles. In yoga exercise, stretching is an integral part of each movement. Cats are a wonderful example of stretching, and their level of suppleness is second to none in the animal kingdom.

Yoga is a gentle exercise system which is believed to encourage union of your body, mind and spirit, and restore balance in three ways. It relaxes your muscles and improves suppleness, fitness and physical function. It relaxes your mind, and shows you how to control stress and destructive emotions. It needs to be practised regularly to have a lasting effect and is taught in classes lasting from one to two hours.

WHAT HAPPENS IN A CLASS?

Classes vary in structure, but in a 90-minute class you would usually begin by focusing on breath control for about 10 minutes, followed by 15–20 minutes of gentle warm-up exercises. It takes time to master the postures – the teacher will reassure you about your level of achievement and encourage you not to push yourself too hard. Postures are usually performed for about 25 minutes, followed by 20 minutes of relaxation exercises. The class may end with 5–10 minutes of reflection, and advice to practise at home in a warm, quiet and well-ventilated room.

Pranayama

This breathing exercise should leave you feeling deeply relaxed. When you exhale, imagine that any feelings of negativity are leaving your mind and body along with your breath.

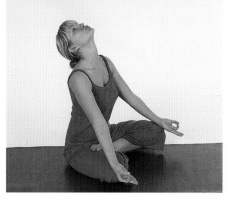

2 Open your mouth to exhale and make a swooshing sound as you exhale the breath.

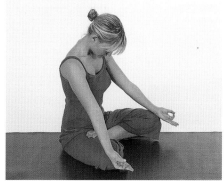

3 Continue to exhale until you drop your chin into your chest.

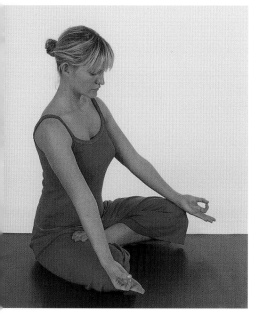

1 Sit up tall in a cross-legged position, half lotus, or full lotus position. It is important that your tailbone touches the floor. Open your palms so they face upwards and place your thumbs and first fingers together. Keep the remaining fingers together and rest the backs of your hands on your knees. Drop your head slightly forwards and gaze at your fingertips. Take a deep inhalation through your nose and slowly take your head all the way back.

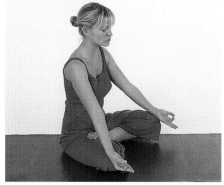

4 Bring your head up and continue to inhale and exhale through your nose for 10 counts. Keep the breath deep and even. Repeat 5 times.

Massage

Three thousand years ago, the wealthy citizens of Greece and Rome began every day with an experience called 'the bath'. For several hours in the early morning they devoted themselves to body care. They either bathed themselves or were bathed by attendants. Intricate exercise programmes were developed to strengthen their bodies, while especially stiff muscles were rubbed with warm oils. A full body massage under the hands of skilful slaves awoke the nerves, stimulated the sluggish blood and freed the action of the joints. Finally, the entire body was rubbed with a fine oil to keep the skin elastic and supple all through the day.

The two-hour morning bath has been replaced in our advanced civilization with a five-minute experience called the shower. This is a pity because, on its most basic level, massage is therapeutic simply because it is an intensely pleasurable experience. The desire to touch and be touched is one of our strongest instincts: we touch each other to show love, to offer security, but also to make us feel better. We can exist without many things but physical contact is not one of them.

Apart from the brain, the skin is the body's most complex organ. Each square centimetre of it contains hundreds of receptors sensitive to touch, pain, pressure, heat and cold.

The basis of modern massage was developed by a Swedish gymnast turned therapist called Professor Per Henrik Ling (1776–1839). He formulated the principles of what became known as Swedish massage.

Today, massage can be found in therapy rooms, beauty salons, homes, sports clubs and hospitals.

THE CONSULTATION

Your first appointment will normally begin with the therapist writing down details about:

- why you have come
- your current state of health
- your medical history
- details of any medication you take
- general lifestyle.

You will be asked to undress, normally in privacy, and lie on the massage table. The therapist will cover you with a towel, and only uncover the parts of your body on which she or he needs to work.

The therapist might massage your back, work down your body, then ask you to turn over and work down your front, paying particular attention to knotty or tense areas. The massage should be relaxing, although you may feel pain in tense areas. You should not feel severe pain – speak out if this happens.

Everyone reacts differently to the treatment: you may feel relaxed, energized, slightly tired, or ache a little the next day. You might cry during the session – this is not unusual if you have been bottling up feelings.

A massage can help you to feel relaxed.

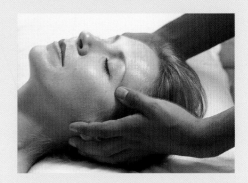

Massage for menopause

There are trigger points within the abdominal wall that, when treated, can bring relief to menopausal symptoms. Here is a massage you can ask a friend or partner to do.

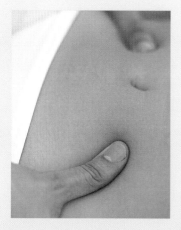

1 Place the pads of your thumbs about 7cm (3in) on either side of the navel and, using your body weight, lean in towards the navel and hold for 5 seconds. Repeat 2–3 times.

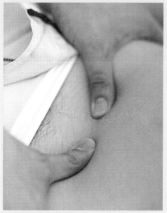

2 Move your thumbs close together and, using the pads, work as in step 1 downwards in a straight line, from just below the navel to end level with the hips. Then work back up, finishing with your thumbs about 7cm (3in) on either side of the navel.

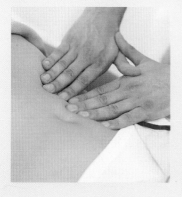

3 Using very light strokes and your hands relaxed and close together, place them on the mid-abdomen, level with the navel, and stroke gently towards the groin and return. Make sure that you massage both sides of the abdomen equally.

WHAT DIFFERENCE COULD MASSAGE MAKE TO MY STRESSFUL LIFE?

Basic massage techniques such as stroking, kneading, wringing, pummelling and knuckling will stimulate your physical and emotional release in two ways – by a mechanical and a reflex action.

The mechanical effects of massage

The mechanical effects are the physical results of pressing, squeezing and moving the soft tissue. This can be either deeply relaxing or stimulating.

For instance, your muscular tension can cause sluggish circulation because it forces your body's blood vessels to constrict. Massaging the muscles frees up such tension and stimulates the circulation so that the blood flows freely, carrying oxygen and nutrients to where they are needed. It can help to normalize blood pressure, easing the pressure on arteries and veins.

Massage also stimulates the lymphatic system, encouraging it to carry waste products out of the body more efficiently and defending it against infection.

The reflex action

The reflex action is an involuntary response of one part of your body to the stimulation of another. Because your body, mind and emotions form one intricate organism, connected by energy channels and a complex nervous system with receptors in the skin, stimulus in one part of your body can affect several other parts. For example, a relaxing back massage can also ease leg pain.

The four stages of healing

There are four stages in the healing process:

1 *Relief*
   The first few treatment sessions will relieve your pain, reduce tension and sedate stressed nerves. They may not necessarily solve your problems, but will ease the symptoms so that you feel better.

2 *Correction*
   The therapist can now work on the underlying cause to prevent the return of the problem. Correctional work could include retuning muscles, decongesting a sluggish lymph system or freeing up fibres that are knotted or scarred.

3 *Strengthening*
   This is important if you have a badly damaged area. Massage can strengthen the surrounding tissues, enabling them to provide adequate support when your injury has healed.

4 *Maintenance*
   Your therapist may recommend a regular check-up, much as dentists do.

THE POWER OF MASSAGE

In 1990 a study was carried out on 30 surgical patients at St Mary's Hospital, London, in connection with pain relief and insomnia. The patients were massaged on the back, face or feet and were then monitored for any physical or psychological changes. Most reported relief from pain, anxiety and muscle spasm, as well as improved sleep and general well-being.The two nurses who performed the massage also reported a better rapport with their patients.

Self-massage at work

When you are menopausal, a good way of combating feelings of stress, irritability and anxiety is to take regular breaks during your working day. Here is a simple routine that can be done while you are at work – all you need is a stable surface and a little time. Repeat each movement as many times as you feel necessary in the time you have available – whether you spend 5 minutes or 20 minutes working on yourself, you will definitely feel the benefit and have more energy for the rest of the day. This routine is particularly good for relieving neck tension, which often causes headaches or a feeling of stiffness.

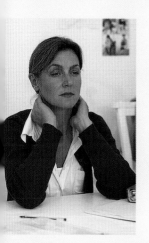

1 Resting your elbows on the desk, place your fingers at the back of your neck behind your ears, leaning your head forward slightly. When you are comfortable, work the length of your neck on either side of the vertebrae by rotating your fingers and applying pressure at the same time.

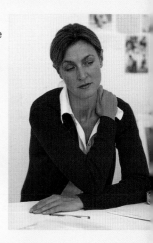

2 Place one hand on the desk and the other on the opposite shoulder. Tilting your head slightly away from the area you are massaging, squeeze the muscle between the fingers and heel of your hand, working from the base of your neck to the edge of your shoulder.

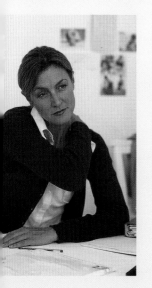

3 In the same position as for step 2, place your fingers on the top of the shoulder muscle and rotate the pads of your fingers while applying pressure, again working from the base of the neck to the edge of the shoulder. Move to the other side and repeat steps 2 and 3.

4 To complete the massage, take the lobe of your ear between your thumb and index finger, close your eyes and visualize a calming scene – a walk along a beach, perhaps. Take a deep breath, and on the out breath pull downwards and off very slowly. Have a drink of water and you will now feel ready to continue your work.

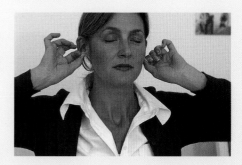

Reflexology

Feet and hands, two hard-working parts of the body, have always been popular sites for massage. The origins of reflexology evidently reach back to Ancient Egypt, as evidenced by a wall carving in the tomb of the renowned doctor Ankmahor which shows doctors working on their patients' hands and feet.

Doctors in Japan, India and China developed their own methods of foot therapy, and this knowledge of Eastern therapies may have been brought to the West by adventurers such as Marco Polo, who wrote that he much admired the Chinese health system.

Reflexology as we know it today was developed in the twentieth century by an American doctor, William Fitzgerald, an ear, nose and throat specialist at Boston General Hospital, using the principles enshrined in zone therapy. According to zone therapy, the body is divided into ten vertical zones, running from the tips of the toes to the top of the head and back down to the fingertips, and all the parts of the body within one zone are linked. By applying pressure to one part of the body, Dr Fitzgerald found it was possible to relieve pain in other areas within the same zone.

Nowadays, zone therapy relies solely on the zones to determine the area to be worked, whereas reflexology takes the zones as well as the anatomical model to determine the area or areas to be worked.

THE CONSULTATION

Your first appointment will probably last for about 90 minutes, and you will be asked about yourself and why you have come for treatment.

- Details of your medical history will be needed, including childhood illnesses, accidents or operations.
- You will need to tell the therapist if you are under the care of a doctor or receiving drug treatment for any illness or chronic (long-term) condition.
- You will be asked how you feel about yourself and your life – your work and leisure activities, as well as your eating, drinking and lifestyle habits.

You will be asked to remove your shoes and socks or tights, and to sit down in a reclining chair or lie on a treatment couch. Your feet may be wiped with some cottonwool soaked in witch hazel, followed by an application of either cream or talcum powder.

First one foot, and then the other, will be worked over by applying pressure to points on them, before giving attention to any problem areas. If you feel pain or tenderness in any area, this is an indication of a blockage or imbalance in the corresponding organ or body part. The intention is not to cause you pain, but pain is a sign of blocked energy – this can be indicated by crystalline deposits under the skin, which can feel like grains of sugar, or the reflexes can be taut or particularly spongy.

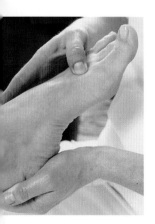

To give a reflexology treatment, a therapist mainly uses her thumb, or sometimes her finger, to apply pressure to different points in order to release any blockage.

Techniques used by the reflexologist may include the following:

- **Thumb walking** This is done with the pad of the thumb, which is pressed into the reflex points. After a few seconds, some of the pressure is released, the thumb slides along (like a caterpillar), stops and then presses again.
- **Finger walking** Similar to thumb walking, except that it is done with the side of the index finger, using the thumb and other three fingers for support.
- **Rotating** The thumb is pressed and rotated into the reflex point.
- **Flexing** The toes are held in one hand while pressure is applied with the thumb of the other hand. The foot is then bent gently backwards and forwards, so that the thumb presses and then releases the point in a rhythmic fashion.

No one knows exactly how reflexology works beyond the physical act of stimulating nerve endings in the feet. We know that there are 70,000 of these nerve endings on the sole of each foot which, when stimulated, can send messages along the pathways of the autonomic nervous system to all areas of the body and brain. By applying pressure to a particular point, known as a reflex point or area, the therapist can stimulate or rebalance the energy in the related zone.

CAN IT HELP MY HOT FLUSHES?

Reflexology works well for any conditions that need to be cleared or regulated, such as menstrual irregularities. If you consult a reflexologist for menopausal symptoms, it is likely that your feet will be worked all over, with special attention paid to the endocrine glands, and the therapist will end by pressing the solar reflex on both feet.

PROVING A POINT

In a randomized controlled study in the USA undertaken in 1993, ear, hand or foot reflexology or a placebo treatment (treating inappropriate reflex zones, too roughly or too lightly) was given to 35 women suffering from PMS. Each woman kept a symptom diary for two months before, during and after eight half-hour reflexology treatments. Thirty-nine symptoms were assessed on a four-point scale. The women given reflexology treatments showed a 46 per cent reduction in the PMS symptoms and discomfort – the placebo group had only a 25 per cent reduction demonstrated.

Reflexology for menopause

This treatment works on the reproductive and endocrine systems, including the thyroid, to help you through the menopause.

1 Find the thyroid reflex point, located on the top of the foot at the base of the big toe. Using your index finger, hook in and press this point for 5 seconds.

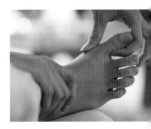

2 Gently work your foot in the area between the back of the heel and the ankle bone. Gently walk all four fingers up to the ankle bone. Find the ovary point and press for 5 seconds.

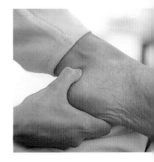

Aromatherapy

If you have enjoyed a full body massage, then your pleasure may be enhanced by the addition of essential oils used by practitioners of aromatherapy. These oils are aromatic essences extracted from plants, flowers, trees, fruit, bark, grasses and seeds. About 150 essential oils have been extracted, each with its own unique scent and healing properties.

All essential oils contain antiseptic properties: some have particular ones that make them antiviral, anti-inflammatory, pain-relieving, antidepressant and expectorating. Others are stimulating, relaxing, aid digestion or have diuretic properties.

Research indicates that the scent of essential oils can exert specific therapeutic effects on our minds and emotions. The oil

An oil burner will release the scent of essential oils into the air, providing natural fragrance while distributing their theraputic benefits.

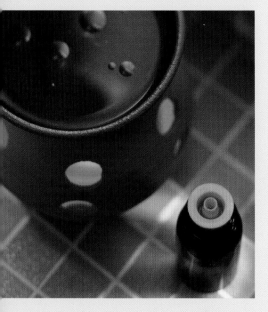

molecules are so small that they can be absorbed through the pores of the skin, affecting the skin itself, the bloodstream and the whole body, including the brain. Heat also helps their absorption, either through warm hands in a massage or from hot bath water.

THE CONSULTATION

Your first appointment with an aromatherapist will last between one and one-and-a-half hours. As with all forms of holistic therapy, the therapist will need to know:

- about you – your medical history and why you have come
- which oils would be best to use, but also those which should be avoided. Some oils are not safe to use if you have blood pressure problems, are epileptic or have had a recent operation
- if you are taking any medicines – or homoeopathic remedies, as strong smells can negate the effects of the latter
- what mood you are in and what kind of day you have had.

You will be asked to undress and lie down on the massage table with a towel over you (you need not undress completely if you feel uncomfortable doing so).

The therapist will leave the towel over you and move it as she or he works around your body – that way you can stay warm and also feel less exposed.

The aromatherapist might decide on a blend of oils thought to suit you, or you may be asked if there are any oils of which you are particularly fond. Then, with this blend of oils, the therapist will begin your massage which will last about 30–45 minutes.

The combination of touch and the therapeutic benefits of the oils improves circulation and releases trapped energy from the muscles. The fragrance also promotes feelings of well-being. For maximum benefit, you may be asked not to bath or shower for a few hours after the massage so that the oils are absorbed thoroughly and completely.

Once they have done their work, the oils will leave your body in various ways: some are exhaled or excreted in urine and faeces, while others are sweated out of your system. The process can take up to six hours in a healthy person, but up to 14 hours in someone who is unhealthy or seriously overweight.

ESSENTIAL OILS FOR MENOPAUSE

Bergamot is excellent for anxiety, depression and stress. It is also a cleansing tonic for the uterus.

Cypress has a calming effect on the mind, soothing anger and frustration.

Clary sage can be used for menstrual problems, depression and anxiety.

Fennel is good for menopausal problems such as irregular periods, pre-menstrual tension and low sexual response.

Geranium is useful for PMT, menopausal problems and anxiety.

Lavender is good for insomnia and headaches.

You can use aromatherapy solutions at home too.

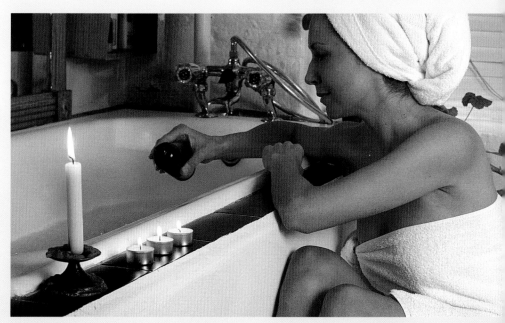

4

Diet

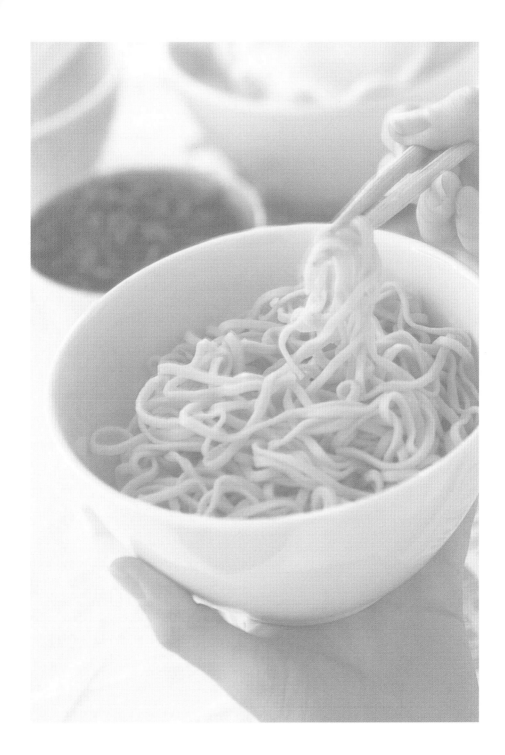

Your diet and the menopause

One of the most important ways that you can stay healthy and energetic in your menopausal years and beyond is to pay close attention to the food you eat. A well-balanced diet that is high in complex carbohydrates, calcium and plant oestrogens, and low in saturated fat and sugar, will go a long way to keeping you slim and healthy and also easing the symptoms of

Cycling can be fun when away from crowded cities and is excellent exercise, whatever your age.

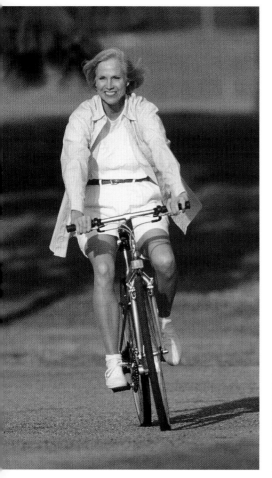

the menopause. If you've often thought about making changes to your dietary habits, now is the time to act. The changes you make to your diet now will determine not only how long you live, but how well you live.

A QUESTION OF BALANCE

Perhaps you think you have maintained a healthy eating lifestyle while cooking for your family, but you are alarmed to discover that a dress you bought a couple of years ago doesn't fit – is this middle-age spread?

Taking stock of your eating and drinking habits now will stand you in good stead for the rest of your life. This does not mean giving up food and drink you enjoy, but recognizing how you can benefit by introducing exciting new perspectives to it as well as modifying some of the less helpful ingredients.

As a child some 60 years ago, the food and drink I consumed was basic, nutritious, wholesome – and predictable. I recall wholemeal bread, meat and two veg, rice pudding and lots of milk. Today, the impact of foreign trade and travel is reflected in the food we buy: pizzas, curries, vast ranges of pastas, sauces, cereals, cheeses, fish, meat and exotic fruits and vegetables – all stimulate our taste buds and empty our wallets. Theoretically, Western society is now better fed than ever before. The reality is that many of us live in a 'toxic food environment' of cheap fatty food, pervasive food advertising and sedentary lives.

> 'Tell me what you eat: I will tell you what you are'
>
> (*Jean-Anthelme Brillat-Savarin, 1825*)

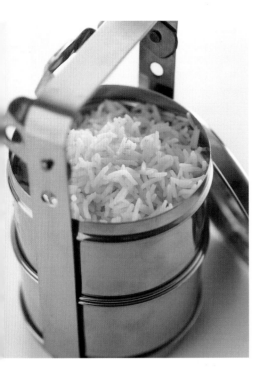

Steaming your food preserves all the vitamins which are often lost in conventional cooking.

Added to which, however confident we are about our choice of diet, warnings constantly appear in the media about the dangers of certain foods, yet statements extolling their virtues are as likely to hit the headlines in the future. So, how do we sort fact from fiction?

BACK TO BASICS

Your body needed nutrients to maintain your physical, mental and emotional well-being from when you were in your mother's womb. As you developed from babyhood, essential nutrients determined your growth:

- Carbohydrates
- Protein
- Fats

Carbohydrates

Carbohydrates are your body's main source of energy for all its functions. They exist in all vegetables, fruits, starches and grains and, in its purest form, in refined sugar.

There are two types of carbohydrates – complex and simple. Complex carbohydrates give a slow release of energy, because it takes time for our digestive tracts to break them down into the simplest substances that our bodies can use. Simple carbohydrates are best avoided where possible: they will make your blood sugar curve rise steeply as a lot of sugar is pumped quickly into your system. The curve is then forced to drop off quickly, so that after a couple of hours your energy levels will plummet and you will feel hungry again.

Complex carbohydrates
- Grains – wheat, rye, oats, rice, barley and maize
- Beans – lentils, kidney beans, chickpeas
- Vegetables
- Fibre in grains, beans and vegetables

Simple carbohydrates
- Fruit, honey, white and brown sugar, and glucose in high-energy drinks

You may be surprised to see fruit described as a 'simple' carbohydrate. Fruit (and honey) contain fructose (also called fruit sugar) which is a simple sugar, but the fibre content of the fruit is a complex carbohydrate that slows the digestion rate. Fructose is fine when taken in whole fruits, like apples and pears, but not when used in the refined form of powdered white sugar.

Proteins

Proteins are found in their largest concentrations in animal foods such as meat, fish, poultry, eggs and cheese, vegetables, foods such as nuts and seeds, and in high-protein legumes such as beans.

Fats

There is more confusion about dietary fat than almost anything else. It is seen as the villain of our eating habits, responsible for weight gain and its ensuing sluggish metabolism. We have all read about low-fat diets and no-fat diets – indeed, many of us have tried them. Sorting out fact from fiction about the nature of fats will help you determine how much you should increase/decrease its inclusion in your diet.

Basically, there are two types of fat – saturated and unsaturated.

Saturated fat

This is found in meat, dairy products like cheese, ice-cream and milk, and tropical oils like palm kernel oil and coconut. If you eat too many foods full of saturated fats they will do their best to lay themselves down as fat stores – hence the connection between fat intake and hardening of the arteries (see page 45).

Olives and olive oil are an excellent source of omega-3 essential fatty acids.

(see page 45)

PROSTAGLANDINS
Beneficial prostaglandins (hormone-like regulating substances) are made by our bodies from omega-3 oils. These prostaglandins are particularly useful at the time of menopause as they help lower blood pressure and decrease sodium (salt) and water retention.

Unsaturated fat

This is a group of fats that includes those called essential fatty acids (EFAs). These are essential for our health: they are a vital component of every human cell and our bodies need them to insulate our nerve cells, keep our skin and arteries supple, balance our hormones and keep us warm.

Unsaturated fat comes in two forms: mono-unsaturates, like olive oil, and poly-unsaturates, found in corn, sunflower seeds and peanuts. Within this group there is a further division into omega-3 and omega-6 fatty acids.

Omega-3 fatty acids

The most important of these is alpha-linolenic acid, found in fish oils and linseed oil, walnuts, pumpkin seeds and dark green vegetables.

Oily fish, such as mackerel, contain oils that can help prevent the onset of heart disease.

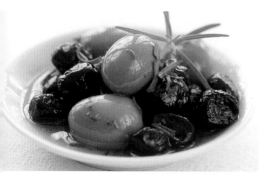

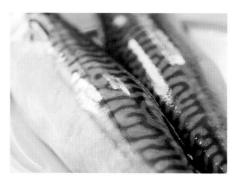

Omega-6 fatty acids

The most important of these is linolenic acid, found in unrefined safflower, corn, sesame and sunflower oils.

Our bodies can make all the fat needed for our daily metabolic processes except for these two essential fatty acids.

The essential fatty acid linolenic acid is converted to gamma-linolenic acid (GLA) which is found in evening primrose oil. Great claims have been made for the powers of evening primrose oil, especially for its success in treating PMS, and it is popularly believed to suppress menopausal flushing.

EFAs can be found in the following:

- Cold-pressed unrefined vegetable oils such as sesame and sunflower oil for salad dressing
- Extra-virgin olive oil for cooking
- Oily fish such as mackerel and sardines
- Nuts (almonds, pecans, brazils) and seeds (sesame, pumpkin, sunflower)
- Tahini (creamed sesame seeds) for sauces and dressings
- Butter in moderation for spreading or for cooking

ON THE GO ALL THE TIME

Pause for a moment and look at your body – it is relaxed and still. What you cannot see is that the inside of it is an energy machine, never resting, always metabolically alive. This machine powers its operations mainly through the use of a basic sugar molecule called glucose. Your body must have glucose, and even under conditions of starvation, it will continue to obtain it as long as there is anything in your body that it can convert into glucose. All of the food you eat is broken down into glucose via the digestive system, and is absorbed through the wall of the intestines into the bloodstream. Once that happens, you then have a high level of glucose in your blood, and your blood sugar levels are said to be high.

As blood glucose rises

As your blood sugar levels go up, which they do after eating simple carbohydrates, such as a bar of chocolate, your body has to make an instant decision – how much of that pure energy should be used for immediate needs and how much should be stored for future requirements?

The instrument for this decision is the hormone insulin, produced by the pancreas, because insulin governs the chemistry of sugar in the body. A rise of sugar in the blood elicits a swift response from insulin, which quickly converts part of this glucose to glycogen, a starch that can be stored in muscles and the liver and can be made readily available to be used as energy.

But what happens if all these glycogen areas are full, and there is still more glucose in the blood than is needed? In this case, insulin stimulates the conversion of the excess glucose to fat molecules called triglycerides: these are part of the overall profile of fats in the body and are frequently elevated in sufferers of heart disease and diabetes.

The roller-coaster glucose ride

Sadly, all those delicious sweet cakes, chocolates and cookies that make our taste buds drool are full of ingredients that are refined. This means that the flour, for example, has been finely processed, and the outer bran of the seed discarded. Most of the fibre is also removed. Fibre absorbs water and contributes to the growth of beneficial bacteria in your gut. This process makes a bulky stool, providing exercise for your bowel and keeping your intestine in healthy working order.

When you eat foods high in such refined ingredients, digestion is very fast and glucose enters your body rapidly, causing your blood sugar levels to rise steeply. In addition, any food or drink that contains a stimulant, such as coffee, tea, alcohol or chocolate, causes a sharp and rapid rise in blood glucose, which may make you feel temporarily more energetic. However, the effect is short-lived. Blood sugar levels soon slump again because simple carbohydrates are unable to maintain them.

When this happens, we feel tired and put on the kettle to make a cup of tea or coffee, then eat a chocolate biscuit – hey presto! – we are revived, full of energy once more. But this boost has caused our blood sugar level to go up rapidly, so repeating the cycle of blood sugar swings. Over time, this roller-coaster stimulation exhausts the pancreas, so that it becomes unable to produce sufficient insulin to regulate blood sugar levels. The result is that too much glucose stays in the blood, instead of being converted into energy or body fat.

If we have not eaten for three hours, our blood glucose will drop to quite a low level, so we again look for the quick boost. At the same time, our adrenal glands will make our livers produce more glucose. The combination of these two causes high levels of glucose in our blood, which again calls on the pancreas to over-produce insulin in order to reduce the glucose levels. The roller-coaster ride starts all over again and our adrenal glands become exhausted because of repeated stimulation.

Why is a steady blood sugar level so important during menopause?

There are many reasons why it is important to avoid the roller-coaster effect on blood sugar levels described above. Maintaining a steady blood sugar level can make a huge difference to how you feel emotionally and physically before, during and after the menopause. Its imbalance puts you at risk of diabetes. And it is especially important during the menopausal years because of the effect on the adrenal glands. As described earlier (page 11), these glands convert androstenadione into oestrone, which will be the main source of oestrogen after the menopause. They also produce a hormone called dehydroepiandrosterone (DHEA) which has been linked to anti-ageing. It is therefore crucial that the adrenal glands are working to their optimum.

Since the maintenance of steady blood sugar levels is such an important factor during the menopause, it clearly makes sense to modify or change your intake of food and drink accordingly. This will be of benefit not only at this time but for the rest of your life.

LOOKING EAST

In Japan, China and Indonesia women so rarely experience hot flushes that their languages do not have words for this menopausal symptom. On the other hand, eight out of ten American women reportedly experience what are termed 'power surges' or 'hot flashes'.

The explanation for this discrepancy, experts say, can be found in diet. The typical diet in the Far East is high in soy and, in Japan, low in processed and refined foods and high in mineral-rich seaweed and fresh fish oils. Not only do Japanese women eating a traditional diet have fewer incidences of hot flushes – they also have lower rates of breast cancer.

The rate of reported menopausal symptoms is also lower in other Asian women, although this could be attributed to a culture that raises its women to 'Never complain, never explain'. It has been noted that when Asian women move to the West and assume a Western diet, then they rapidly develop the diseases encountered there.

RECENT CHINESE STUDY

The China Diet Study began gathering information on the lifestyles of 6,500 adults in 1983. One hundred people from each of the 65 provinces comprising China answered 367 questions about their diets, lives and bodies. This ten-year study is the most comprehensive study ever conducted on the eating habits of Chinese people.

It was an exacting, labour-intensive study, initially financed by the US National Cancer Institute, that could probably not have been done anywhere except China. Nowhere else is there a genetically similar population with such great regional differences in disease rates, dietary habits and environmental exposures. And nowhere else could researchers afford to hire hundreds of trained workers to carry out the investigation. Three days were spent in each household, collecting blood and urine samples and gathering exact information on what and how much people ate. Food samples were also analysed for their nutrient contents.

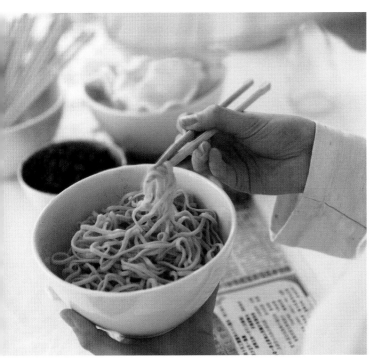

Far Eastern food is often low in processed and refined ingredients.

It was money well spent, for it has turned out to be a very important study – unique and well done, and one that challenges much of dietary dogma. Highlights of this 920 page study show that:

- Chinese people consume 20 per cent more calories than Americans do, but Americans are 25 per cent heavier. This is because the Chinese eat three times the amount of starch and only one-third the amount of fat. This is a more important factor than exercise.
- Cholesterol levels in China are much lower than in the USA. The Chinese average is 127 mg/dL, compared with 212 mg/dL in the USA.
- Protein intake in China is one-third less than in the USA – 64 g (2¼ oz) per person per day, compared with 100 g (3½ oz).
- While Chinese women eat only half the calcium that American women eat, osteoporosis is uncommon in China. Most Chinese people eat no dairy products at all and obtain their calcium from plant foods.

Japanese diets are often high in seaweed, which is rich in minerals.

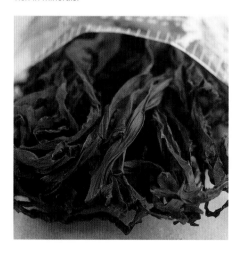

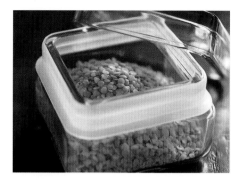

Legumes, such as lentils, contain phyto-oestrogens.

- In China, mortality rates resulting from colon cancer are lowest where cholesterol levels are lowest.
- For every heart attack in China, there are 16 in the USA.
- Female cancers relate to diet. A childhood diet high in protein, fat, calcium and calories promotes rapid growth and early onset of menstruation. This increases a woman's risk for developing cancer of the reproductive organs and the breast. Chinese women rarely get these cancers and they begin menstruating 3–6 years later than American women.
- The Chinese diet is three times richer in fibre than a typical Western one, resulting in relatively low rates of colon cancer.
- Iron-deficiency anaemia is rare in China, though their diet is mainly plant food and they eat less meat than in the West. The average Chinese adult consumes twice the iron the average American does, but the vast majority of it comes from plants.

SOY FAR, SO GOOD

Some plants contain substances that, when eaten, can affect hormone status. These substances are called phyto-oestrogens. Perhaps the most famous example of this is the soya bean. Soya beans contain phyto-oestrogens known as isoflavones, which make up about 75 per cent of the soya protein. In the human gut, enzymes convert these into compounds that can have an oestrogenic action, even though they are not hormones. Although the potencies are considerably weaker than the oestrogen produced by the ovaries (estradiol), they appear to mimic and modulate oestrogens and can help to stabilize hormone fluctuations. Depending on the tissue and the concentration, phyto-oestrogens either act as hormones or they inhibit the actions of natural hormones. In this way, they may do a similar job to tamoxifen (the breast cancer drug), which binds on to oestrogen receptors and inhibits breast cancer growth.

Foods that contain phyto-oestrogens include the following:

- Wholegrains (such as wheat, corn and oats)
- Legumes (such as chickpeas, mung beans, lentils and peas)
- Garlic
- Linseed
- Sunflower and pumpkin seeds
- Almonds, cashews and peanuts
- Radishes
- Potatoes
- Fennel
- Celery
- Sprouting beans (such as alfalfa)
- Parsley
- Green tea
- Papaya
- Rhubarb
- Apples

However, it is the soy products like tofu (soya bean curd), tempeh, miso, tamari (wheat-free soy sauce made in the traditional way), natto, okara and yuba, as well as soya milk and soya protein powder, which are the simplest ways to incorporate phyto-oestrogens into your meals. A recommended daily dose of 45 g (1½ oz) of soy protein has been found to reduce hot flushes by 40 per cent.

SOY-EXTRACT TABLETS

Soy products are very much an acquired taste for many Westernized palates. If you find them unpleasant, try soya-extract tablets twice daily for a few months.

RED CLOVER ISOFLAVONE

In double-blind controlled trials, systemic arterial compliance (a measure that correlates with less risk of CVD) was significantly improved in women taking a red clover isoflavone supplement, and the rate of bone density loss in peri-menopausal women taking the same supplement was halved over a 12-month period.

A SLICE OF GOOD FORTUNE

Nearly 20 years ago, a woman living in Yorkshire, England, made a momentous decision, little knowing what would develop from it. Linda Kearns had been on hormone replacement therapy for 13 years following a hysterectomy and oophorectomy (removal of ovaries) but had never really felt 100 per cent. She always felt tired and a little under the weather. Following a breast cancer scare, she decided enough was enough and stopped taking HRT. Her hot flushes and night sweats reappeared overnight.

She began reading up about alternative remedies, and discovered she could replace the HRT using foods rich in phyto-oestrogens. The problem was that some natural seeds and grains on their own are rather unappetising, so Linda set about creating a tasty cake.

Keeping flushes away

Within three weeks of starting to eat the resulting cake, her menopausal symptoms disappeared and she was bursting with energy. She now eats two slices of her cake every day at breakfast and after her evening meal.

When word got out, she found herself inundated with a request for the recipe (see right). Today, upwards of 2,000 of these cakes (available in raisin, cherry and cranberry), are baked every day at a Yorkshire bakery.

About 100 g (4 oz) a day (or a third of a 300 g (11 oz) cake) is usually adequate to deliver sufficient phyto-oestrogens to relieve menopausal symptoms. A 100 g (4 oz) slice looks generous, but it does not have to be eaten all at once. And you don't need to worry about the sugar and fat content: there are no added fats other than those naturally occurring in the various seeds, and no added sugar.

Recipe for the Linda Kearns Cake

Ingredients
100 g (4 oz) soya flour
100 g (4 oz) wholewheat flour
100 g (4 oz) porridge oats
100 g (4 oz) linseeds
50 g (2 oz) sunflower seeds
50 g (2 oz) pumpkin seeds
50 g (2 oz) sesame seeds
50 g (2 oz) flaked almonds
2 pieces of stem ginger, finely chopped
200 g (8 oz) raisins
Approx 750 ml (1¼ pt) soya milk
1 tablespoon malt extract
½ teaspoon nutmeg
½ teaspoon cinnamon
½ teaspoon ground ginger

Place the dry ingredients in a large bowl and mix thoroughly, then add the soya milk and malt extract. Mix well and leave to soak for about half-an-hour. (If the mixture is too stiff, add more soya milk.) Spoon into two loaf tins lined with greaseproof paper and oil. Bake in the oven at gas mark 5/190°C/375°F for about 1¼ hours or until cooked through (test with a skewer). Turn out and leave to cool. The cake is delicious with butter or spread. Ideally, eat a slice a day.
Note *The cake is not artificial HRT. It is a cake containing only the ingredients listed, which themselves contain natural plant phyto-oestrogens.*

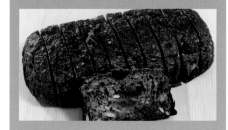

Good health off the shelf

If you read glossy magazines, listen to commercial radio or watch TV, or if you explore the plethora of health websites on the Internet, you will know that there is a thriving industry devoted to the promotion of vitamin and mineral supplements. These are aimed at people concerned about a variety of conditions and, increasingly, combinations of vitamins and minerals are being marketed for specific groups of people, such as menopausal women.

Adverts often feature an amazing display of attractively presented pills, potions and packets, bristling with complicated neo-scientific data on the labels – so how do you decide which, if any of them, will improve or maintain your health?

First of all, you need to know what the various vitamins and minerals actually do in the human body.

VITAMINS

- **Vitamin A** maintains your healthy skin, eyes, bones, hair and teeth.
- **Vitamin D** assists in the absorption and metabolism of calcium and phosphorus for strong bones and teeth.
- **Vitamin E** helps protect your red blood cells, circulation and heart. As an antioxidant, vitamin E helps to protect cell membranes, fats and vitamin A from destructive oxidation.
- **Vitamin K** is needed for proper clotting of your blood and is vital for bone formation.
- **Vitamin C** (ascorbic acid) is important for maintenance of your bones, teeth, collagen (which makes up 90 per cent of our bone matrix) and blood vessels. We neither manufacture nor store our own vitamin C, so we need to make sure that we obtain adequate amounts during the day.

B vitamins

Four of the B group vitamins – B1, B2, B3 and B6 – release energy from the food we eat, as well as performing other functions.

- **Vitamin B1** (thiamine) is needed for a normal appetite and for the functioning of a healthy nervous system.
- **Vitamin B2** (riboflavin) is necessary for healthy skin and eyes.
- **Vitamin B3** (niacin) helps to maintain the skin, nervous system and promotes proper mental functioning.
- **Vitamin B6** plays a role in protein and fat metabolism and is essential for the function of red blood cells.
- **Vitamin B5** (pantothenic acid) fights infections and helps to strengthen the immune system.
- **Vitamin B12** (cobalamin) prevents pernicious anaemia and is necessary for a healthy nervous system.
- **Vitamin B17** (amygdalin) is purported to control cancer.

RED BLOOD CELLS

Red cells float in the blood and are the means by which oxygen reaches all parts of the body. They contain a protein, haemoglobin, which has a special ability to grab oxygen molecules as the cells circulate through the lungs and then release it wherever it is needed in the tissues. Iron is an essential constituent of haemoglobin, and anaemia is the result of lack of haemoglobin.

MINERALS

- **Calcium** protects and builds bones and teeth and aids blood clotting.
- **Chromium** breaks down sugar so it can be used in the body and helps to regulate blood pressure.
- **Iron** aids growth, promotes the immune system and is essential for the metabolism and production of haemoglobin.
- **Manganese** is needed for normal bone structure and is important for both the hormone production of the thyroid gland and for digestion.
- **Magnesium** is extremely important for the health of your bones – equally if not more important than calcium (see box). You need twice as much magnesium as calcium if the biochemistry of your bone formation is to run smoothly.
- **Phosphorus** maintains healthy, strong bones and teeth, and is necessary for muscle and nerve function.
- **Potassium** regulates your body's water balance, aids muscle function and helps to dispose of the body's waste.
- **Selenium** is a trace element that occurs

Spinach is a rich source of iron and vitamin K.

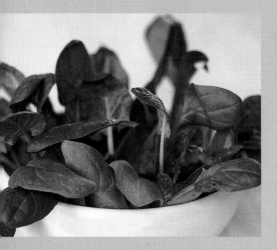

MARVELLOUS MAGNESIUM

Sixty per cent of your body's magnesium stores are contained in your bones, particularly in the trabecular bone of your wrist, thighs and vertebrae. Magnesium is vital in metabolizing calcium and vitamin C, and helps to convert vitamin D to the active form necessary to ensure proper calcium absorption.

naturally in the soil, foods and your body. It is a potent antioxidant, preventing or slowing down ageing, and is vital to activate thyroid hormones and keep your liver functioning healthily.

- **Sulphur** helps to fight bacterial infection, aids your liver and forms part of tissue-building amino acids.
- **Sodium** (salt) is essential for normal growth and helps muscles and nerve function. It is, however, excessive in most people's diets.
- **Zinc** is present in small amounts as a component of insulin and is required for blood sugar control, as well as for hearing and proper taste. It is also important for healing of wounds and assists the activity of vitamin D in promoting the absorption of calcium supplements.

From the chart on pages 104–107, you will be able to check exactly which vitamins and minerals feature in your current diet. Once you have done this, you might realize that you do not eat enough foods containing vitamins B1 or B12, or minerals such as magnesium or potassium, for example, so increasing these with a supplement could be the answer. Equally, you may not like drinking milk or eat much in the way of dairy products, so this chart will show you other foods from which you can gain the calcium you need.

CALCIUM SUPPLEMENTS

If you decide to buy a calcium supplement, look very carefully at the label. Calcium carbonate is the cheapest and most widely marketed calcium supplement – it is otherwise known as chalk. Be aware that calcium carbonate is an inorganic mineral; it is mined from the ground and is not present in this particular form in any plant or animal. It can increase your risk of kidney stones and is not even particularly well absorbed into the body's system. On the other hand, calcium citrate is absorbed well. The following test will show you if the supplement you are taking is being absorbed: place your supplement in a glass of warm vinegar for 30 minutes, stirring every few minutes. The warm vinegar roughly represents the conditions found in your gut. If the supplement does not dissolve after 30 minutes, try another type.

SENSIBLE SUPPLEMENTS

Supplements are regularly dismissed by nutritionists as being unnecessary, but they are the answer if you have neither the time nor inclination to prepare nutritious food for yourself, or you are reassured by taking a tablet that contains a specified daily requirement. There is growing evidence that supplements can have a beneficial effect on menopausal symptoms, especially the following:

- Lambert's Gynovite Plus – multivitamins and minerals for women during and after the menopause. (Recommended by the UK Women's Nutritional Advisory Service.)
- BioCare Isoflavone Complex – fermented soy and vitamins B6 and E. (Biocare products are available in Europe as well as Singapore, South Africa, Israel and Oman.)
- BioCare Phytosterol Complex – natural source of plant sterols.

- Solgar Earth Source – suitable for vegetarians. Solgar has spent several years employing rabbinical supervision to obtain kosher certification – look for the KOF-K symbol on these products. (This supplement is manufactured in the USA and sold in 20 countries worldwide.)

FATTY ACIDS

If you decide to take an appropriate vitamin and mineral preparation, the next most important nutritional group for long-range supplementation is the essential fatty acids. As mentioned earlier in this chapter, they are a vital component of every human cell and your body needs them to:

- insulate your nerve cells
- keep your skin and arteries supple
- balance your hormones, and
- keep you warm.

Linseeds provide a source of omega-3 fatty acids. Biocare's linseed oil (flaxseed oil) is manufactured in either capsule form or lemon-flavoured powder in 500 mg or 1000 mg.

Linseeds can be bought as seeds or as oil.

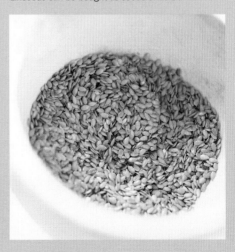

Food fitness

Try to buy high-quality food from good sources and eat:

- Fruits and vegetables – abundantly
- Wholegrains and cereals – moderately
- Beans, peas and lentils – often
- Fats and concentrates (foods that are high in protein, fat or sugar) – sparingly

The following foods are all rich sources of vitamins and minerals.

FRUIT

Apples *iron, manganese, vitamins A, B1, B2, B3, B17, C, D and E*

Apricots *sodium, zinc, vitamin B17*

Avocado *manganese, vitamins B, C and E*

Bananas *potassium, chromium, vitamins B and C*

Blackberries *vitamins B, C and E*

Cherries *vitamins B and C*

Cranberries *vitamin C*

Damsons *vitamins B and E*

Dates *sodium, vitamin B*

Figs *sodium, sulphur, vitamins B and C*

Gooseberries *vitamins B, C and E*

Grapefruit *potassium, phosphorus, vitamins B and C*

Grapes *iron, vitamins B, C and E*

Guavas *vitamin C*

Kiwi fruit *vitamin C*

Lemon *vitamins B and C*

Loganberries *vitamins B and C*

Mangoes *vitamins B and C*

Melons *vitamin C*

Nectarines *zinc, vitamin B17*

Olives *sodium*

Oranges *magnesium, vitamin C*

Papaya *vitamins A, B1, B3 and B5*

Passion fruit *vitamins B and C*

Peaches *manganese, vitamins B and C*

Pineapple *vitamin C*

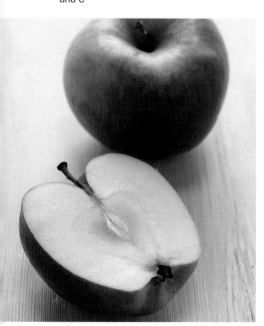

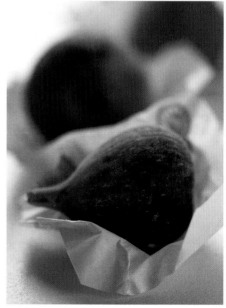

Plums *iron, vitamins B17 and C*
Quince *iron, vitamins B and C*
Raspberries *sodium, sulphur, vitamins B, C and E*
Rhubarb *vitamins B, C and E*
Strawberries *sodium, sulphur, vitamins B and C*
Tangerines *vitamins B and C*
Tomatoes *potassium, vitamins B, C and E*
Ugli fruit (a citrus fruit indigenous to Jamaica, a cross between a grapefruit and a tangerine) *potassium, phosphorus, magnesium, vitamin C*

VEGETABLES

Artichokes *potassium, vitamins A, B and C*
Asparagus *potassium, vitamins A, B, C and E*
Aubergines *magnesium, phosphorus, vitamin B*
Beans *vitamin B12*
Beetroot *vitamin C*

Broccoli *selenium, vitamin E*
Brussels sprouts *sulphur, vitamin C*
Carrots *sulphur, vitamins A, B and C*
Cauliflower *potassium, vitamins B, C and E*
Courgette *vitamins B and E*
Garlic *sulphur, vitamins A, B1,B 2, B3, B5 and C*
Kale *calcium, phosphorus, potassium, sulphur, vitamin A*
Leafy green vegetables *iron, vitamins B2 and C*
Mushrooms *vitamins C and E*
Okra (an African plant, also called gumbo) *magnesium, sulphur, vitamins B and C*
Onions *selenium, sulphur, vitamins B3 and C*
Parsley *vitamins A, B3, B5, and E*
Parsnips *sulphur, vitamins B, C and E*
Peas *calcium, vitamins B and C*
Peppers *vitamin C*
Plantain *vitamins B and C*
Potatoes *calcium, chromium, sulphur, vitamin C*

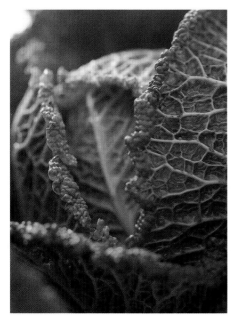
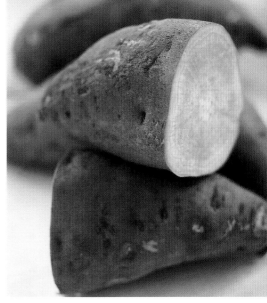

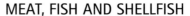

Pumpkin *iron, zinc, vitamins B and C*
Radishes *potassium, vitamin C*
Red cabbage *magnesium, vitamins B and C*
Savoy cabbage *vitamins B, C and E*
Spinach *calcium, iron, chromium, vitamins B, E and K*
Spring cabbage *vitamins B and C*
Spring onions *vitamin C*
Squash *iron, phosphorus*
Sweetcorn *vitamins B and E*
Watercress *vitamins B3, C and D*
White cabbage *vitamins B and C*
Yams (sweet potatoes) *vitamins A, B and C*

DAIRY FOODS

Butter *enjoy occasionally*
Cheese *vitamin B2, enjoy in moderation*
Cream *resist!*
Eggs *sodium, sulphur (egg yolk), zinc, vitamins B2, B12 and E*
Milk *calcium, vitamins B12 and D*
Yogurt *vitamins A, B, D and E*

MEAT, FISH AND SHELLFISH

Bacon *buy the best! Grill rather than fry*
Herring *vitamins B2 and D*
Oysters *zinc, vitamin B*
Quahog (an edible clam) *phosphorus, selenium*
Salmon *calcium, vitamins B2 and D*
Tuna *phosphorus, selenium, vitamins B2 and D*

BEANS

Chickpeas *vitamins C and E*
Soya beans *calcium, potassium*
Soya flour *vitamin B*

SEEDS

Pumpkin seeds *iron, zinc, vitamins B and C*
Sesame seeds *calcium, phosphorus, vitamin B1*
Sunflower seeds *vitamin B1*

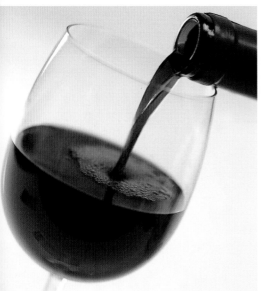

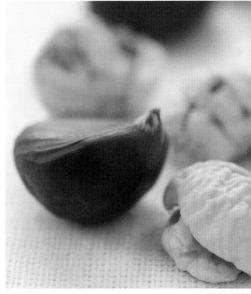

NUTS

Almonds *calcium, magnesium, vitamins B2 and E*

Barcelonas *vitamins B and C*

Brazils *iron, phosphorus, vitamins B and E*

Cashews *magnesium, vitamins B and E*

Chestnuts *potassium, vitamins B and C*

Coconut *sulphur, vitamins B, C and E*

Hazelnuts *vitamins B and E*

Peanuts *vitamins B1 and E*

Pecan *vitamins B and C*

Pinenuts *vitamin B*

Pistachios *vitamin B*

Walnuts *iron, magnesium, vitamins B, C and E*

GRAINS

Bread *The staff of life. (Take care with some white breads as they may contain sugar or dextrose and/or flour improvers – the latter is fine if it states 'ascorbic acid' on the label as this is a form of Vitamin C.)*

Chapatis *vitamin B*

Rye bread *vitamins A, B1, B2, B3, B5, B12 and E, and manganese*

Wholemeal bread *chromium and manganese*

Rice *iron, magnesium, phosphorus, vitamin B1*

CEREALS

(Read the label to check sugar content.)

Bran *selenium, phosphorus, iron, vitamin B1*

Oats *magnesium, sodium, vitamin B1*

Wheatgerm *zinc, magnesium, vitamins B1 and E*

BEVERAGES

Champagne *enjoy!*

Cocoa *zinc, vitamins B and E*

Coffee *reduce*

Tea *manganese, vitamins B and C*

Water *drink 8 glasses a day*

Wine *vitamin B in red wine is excellent for your heart!*

SWEET TREATS AND SAVOURY SNACKS

Biscuits *avoid, they are usually full of refined sugar*

Cakes *resist!*

Chocolate *special treat only!*

Crisps *vitamins B, C and E*

Danish pastries *resist!*

Honey *calcium*

Ice cream *calcium*

Jam *vitamin C*

Peanut butter *vitamins B, C and E*

Sugar *Refined white has no vitamins, demerara and muscavado contain vitamin B*

5
Exercise

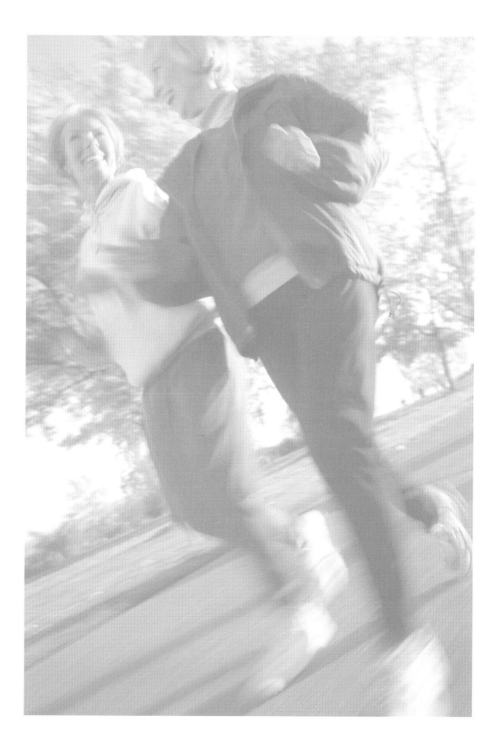

Get moving!

The advantages of regular physical exercise are numerous and well-documented. Exercise allows you to burn fat more efficiently, and it boosts the metabolism so that you continue to burn off calories at a faster rate even after you have stopped exercising, thereby helping to control body weight.

Exercise can have a powerful all-round effect on your health. Regular exercise helps to keep the bowels working efficiently, which gets rid of waste products your body does not need. In addition, it:

- improves the function of the immune and lymph systems, and the ability of the body to keep blood sugar levels in balance
- maintains bone density
- maintains muscle mass
- increases metabolism, burning calories and fat
- reduces stress
- alleviates many menopausal symptoms, such as hot flushes
- helps former smokers stay off cigarettes

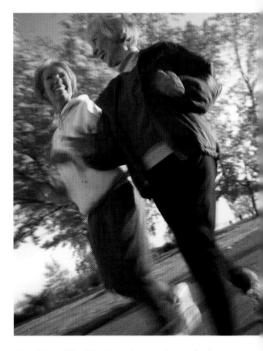

Exercising with a friend can be an extra motivation.

- boosts the immune system, lessening vulnerability to colds and 'flu
- helps maintain flexibility and joint movement as you age.

A HEALTHY HEART

Regular exercise is vital to keep your heart healthy. Research consistently shows that it helps to keep arteries flexible and reduces cholesterol levels.

Aerobic exercise – which speeds up your heart rate – is considered ideal for a healthy heart, so aim for 30 minutes of aerobic activity such as swimming, brisk walking, running or cycling at least three times a week.

Start gently and build up gradually. Mild breathlessness is normal and healthy.

COUNT THE CALORIES

How many calories do you burn off doing everyday activities? This is how much you can use up in 20 minutes:

Activity	Calories burned
Ironing	20
Housework	60
Digging the garden	100
Walking upstairs	120
Running upstairs	200

Keeping up the pressure

Physical activity can help to keep your blood pressure low, and an hour of brisk walking five times a week is recommended for maximum benefit. However, if you don't have time for one long exercise session each day, short bursts of activity that fit into your daily routine can be effective too. Take the stairs instead of the lift, get off the bus a stop early and try to cycle instead of taking the car on short trips.

BUILD BONES AND MUSCLES

Your bones and muscles need weight-bearing exercise to boost bone density. Such high-impact activities include:

- Skipping
- Aerobics
- Tennis
- Running
- Gentle weight-training

EXERCISE YOUR MIND

Your mental health will also benefit from regular exercise. Physical activity releases 'feel-good' endorphins, which boost your mood and help you to relax.

Swimming and jogging can also help to calm your mind, while your mood will be lifted by steps accompanied by music – dancing is guaranteed to 'banish the blues' of a difficult menopause (see page 124).

ENDORPHINS

Endorphins are chemicals secreted by the brain that help us to feel happier, calmer and more alert.

GETTING MOTIVATED

Going to a gym or health fitness centre may suit you and your lifestyle – but it may not. Many of us are put off by the membership fees and the need to buy the right clothes, as well as worrying about our exposure in front of strangers. It is easy to feel intimidated or uncomfortable, and you will soon lose your motivation if you don't enjoy the experience.

But many gyms and leisure centres offer a huge range of possibilities – from salsa and belly dancing to kickboxing and rockclimbing – so it is worth taking the time to investigate what is available.

Swimming is a fun way to exercise.

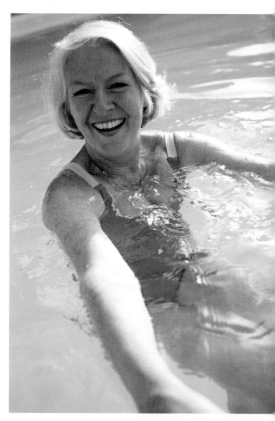

Leg swing

This exercise will improve your flexibility and circulation. Use a cushion if you find your joints are uncomfortable when kneeling on the floor.

1 Kneel on all fours. You can do this exercise with or without small hand weights. If you choose to use them, place one in the bend of your right knee. Lift your lower leg slightly to keep the weight in place.

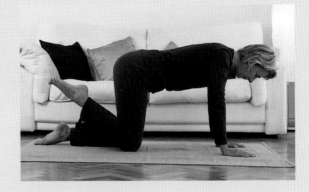

2 Lift the bent knee until it is level with your spine and your right foot is pointing up to the ceiling.

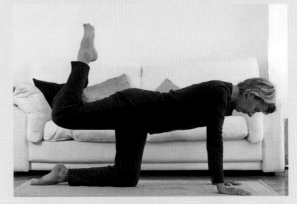

3 Swing your bent leg down and through until your knee is under your chest. Return it to the starting position and lower to the ground. Repeat the exercise using the other leg.

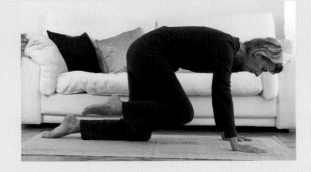

Kneeling hand walk

This exercise places much needed pressure on your hand and arm joints and bones. Make sure that your spine is kept straight by not letting your head hang.

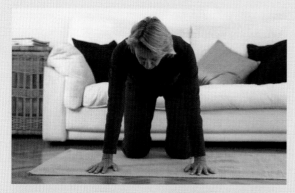

4 Kneel down on all fours, keeping your back straight.

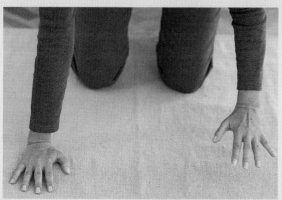

5 Keeping your knees and feet still, slowly walk your hands forward until your arms are carrying the bulk of your weight. Be sure to keep your spine straight.

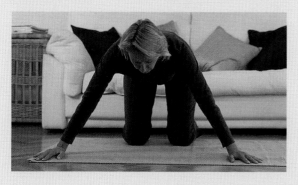

6 Now walk your hands out to the side. This will greatly increase the strength of the bones in your arms. Then walk your hands back in the reverse pattern until you are kneeling comfortably, balanced on all fours again. Repeat this a few times and then stand up.

Posturing with purpose

In childhood we have a naturally relaxed posture, but as we mature our bodies start to reflect the strains of life. It is easy to get into the habit of slouching in a squashy armchair or sitting hunched in front of a computer screen without taking a break. Some jobs necessitate standing for long periods or performing repetitive actions. All these occupations can place undue stress on specific parts of our bodies.

Every day we acquire incorrect posture without noticing that it is happening, and this in turn filters through to other physical functions and depletes our energy.

Other postural problems can have an emotional basis – people who carry an emotional burden can often be seen literally to carry it on their shoulders.

One condition that can be rectified by particular exercises is kyphosis. This curvature of the top of the spine is sometimes associated with osteoporosis, and is therefore frequently seen in post-menopausal women.

If kyphosis is becoming a problem for you, you may find it helpful to make the Pilates system part of your daily routine. This exercise method was formulated by Joseph Pilates, a German gymnast, skier, boxer, wrestler and physical fitness trainer, and is based on the premise that our physical movements most benefit our health when they are conscious actions serving our will. So whether we are walking, sitting, turning or stretching, we should always direct our movements, clear in our minds as to exactly what we are doing and how advantageous it will be to us.

Pilates is different from other forms of exercise primarily because of its holistic approach and its combined training of mind and body to achieve correct alignment.

Its key elements are:

- lengthening short muscles and strengthening weak muscles
- improving the quality of movement
- focusing on the core postural muscles to stabilize the body
- working to place the breath correctly
- controlling even the smallest movements
- understanding and improving good body mechanics
- mental relaxation.

BAD POSTURE   GOOD POSTURE

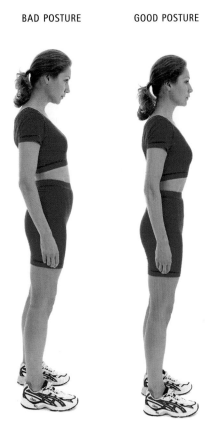

Good posture is not just about having a straight back. It lends balance to our limbs, allowing movements such as walking to be performed more smoothly. We all have our own unique way of walking, and an awareness of your body's posture can add balance and control to what are otherwise unconscious movements, such as standing, sitting and lying.

STANDING

If you watch people standing – say at a bus stop or queuing at a check-out – you will notice how often they simply do not know what to do with their bodies.

They put the weight on one leg, bending the other – then shift their weight to the other leg. There is an attempt to stand up straight, but knees get locked and the pelvis is pushed forward, creating an exaggerated hollow in the lower spine. And as for arms – we do not know what to do with them! They get folded across our bodies, or hands are clasped behind our backs, or we place our hands on our hips. It is as if we have no sense of gravity within our bodies. If we can find it, it will hold us in a position of balance and ease.

How to stand

- Stand with your feet hip-width apart.
- Make sure that both your legs are facing directly forward.
- Your legs need to be straight but your knees should not be locked back into the joint.
- Allow your arms to rest naturally at your sides, falling over the middle of your hips.
- Feel your weight being supported by the middle of each foot.
- Do not rock back, allowing the heels to take your weight, or place your weight on the balls of your feet.

Your confidence will be boosted by a well-balanced body.

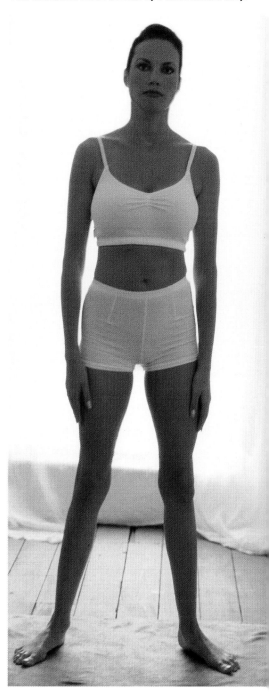

Once you have achieved this way of resting, with your muscles relaxed and your balance centred, you will find that you tire less easily, feel taller and are generally more relaxed in your environment.

SITTING

Like standing, sitting is something we often do not do very well. We sit balanced on one hip bone, then we shift to the other. We cross our legs or sit with one leg underneath us. We wriggle around in our seats, trying to find a position that is comfortable. When we eventually do find a comfortable position, it does not seem to last long.

We try to find external solutions to this, such as lumbar supports on chairs or car seats. The trouble with these is that they are not suitable for most of us – they are too low down to give support where it is needed. Instead, they tend to push the lumbar spine forward, and this in turn can push the abdominal muscles and the internal organs forward.

Choosing a chair

When looking for a chair that will properly support the back and allow you to adopt a good sitting posture, you need to check out the following points:

- You should be able to sit comfortably with your whole thigh supported by the seat of the chair.
- You should be able to place both feet flat on the floor comfortably.
- The back support should be as high as your shoulder blades – the backs of many office chairs are either lower or higher than this.

Remember to sit with your weight evenly distributed, your knees slightly apart in order to support the weight, and your feet together, underneath your knees.

You should be able to place both feet flat when you sit down.

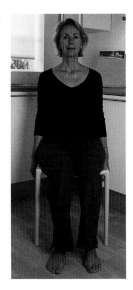

Lying down

We spend approximately one-third of each day lying down. Again, we do not give much thought to this, we just do it, and as we are sleeping for much of this time, we are unaware of our position.

Lying down should be our ultimate position of rest, but still we manage to contort ourselves in various ways that put strain on our muscles and limit our blood circulation. How often have you woken up with stiff muscles and a sore back? Sleeping on your stomach will not support your spine, as it often gets twisted if one leg is bent up when you are in this position. To breathe properly while lying on your stomach, your head has to be turned to one side. This not only twists the neck but can also trap nerves in it, leading to feelings of numbness or 'pins and needles'.

The best positions for sleeping are on your back or side. If you have a lower-back problem, it can be helpful to sleep with a pillow between your knees.

WAKE-UP TIME!

How often do you wake up and instinctively feel like a good stretch even before you put a foot out of bed? Quite often your whole body moves into that stretch, elongating your back, your arms and your legs, but without you consciously willing them. You might even yawn while you do it – another reflex action. Stretching your body like this feels pleasurable, but how good is it for you?

Stretching helps to lengthen your muscles and to relax them. If we think of our muscles as having the same qualities as elastic bands, it is easy to understand the aim of doing stretches. Too much tension tightens our muscles, and makes us feel tired and depressed. Relieving the muscle tension by stretching brings back elasticity and aids muscle/joint harmonization.

Tight muscles cause a number of problems, and as the muscles are interconnected, an injury or condition may not arise in the area of tightness, but instead in an area connected to it. For instance, lower-back injuries can result from tight hamstring muscles at the back of the knees. Tight hamstrings restrict mobility and result in your lower back also being tight. Very tight hamstrings pull on your pelvis, creating postural problems.

Stretching your muscles should feel comfortably uncomfortable. The sensation should be one of stretching, not one of tearing. Take care! If you experience a hot, shooting pain while stretching then stop the exercise immediately, otherwise you are likely to cause yourself damage.

While you sleep you will change your position many times.

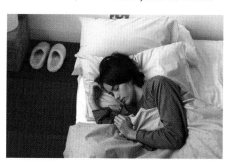
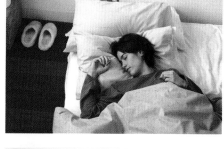
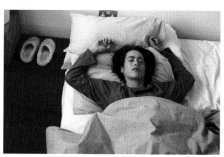
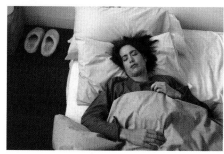

Hamstring stretch

The hamstrings are the two tendons at the rear of the hollows of your knees. Tendons are constructed of tough, inelastic fibrous tissue that connects a muscle with its bony attachment. This Pilates exercise will help you to stretch them.

1 Place your buttocks on the edge of a desk or the arm of a sofa, just enough to support your pelvis. Place the heel of one foot on a low stool in front of you. Make sure that the stool is close enough for you not to have to stretch out your leg to reach it. Turn your foot outwards to stretch your buttock and hamstring muscles.

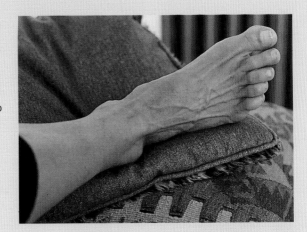

2 Next, turn your foot inwards in order to stretch the inner part of your hamstring.

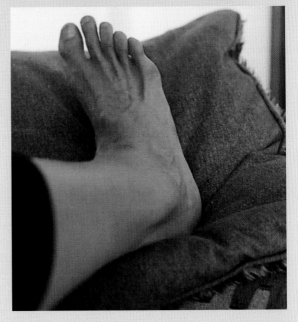

Shoulder stretch

This is a Pilates exercise that will help you to stretch your shoulders. Repeat this exercise 3–6 times.

1 Kneel with a cushion between your knees and calves. Squeeze the cushion and clasp your hands behind your back at the level of your buttocks. Breathe in, pull up your pelvic floor and pull in your stomach muscles.

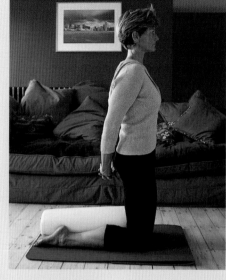

2 Breathe out, pull your shoulders back and squeeze your shoulder blades together.

3 Stretch your clasped hands away from your buttocks. Hold the position for 3 breaths.

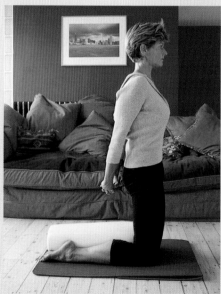

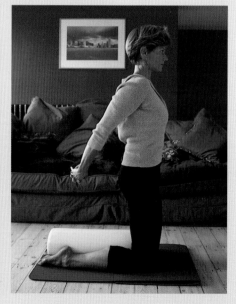

Neck stretch

The aim of this Pilates exercise is to stretch and relax your neck muscles. Repeat each of these steps 1–3 times.

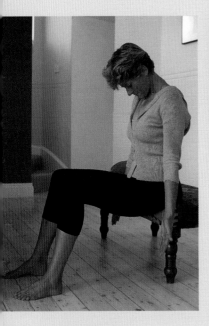

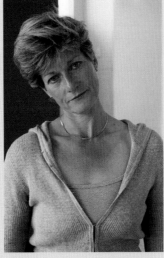

2 Drop your right ear towards your right shoulder as far as it is comfortable. Hold for 10–30 long slow breaths.

1 Sit on the edge of a chair or bed. Tuck your chin in towards your chest. Allow yourself to melt like an ice cube from your chest and stomach muscles, letting the spine drop forwards. Hold the position for 10–30 long slow breaths.

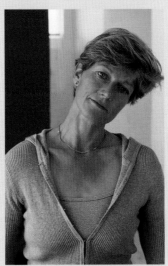

3 Now drop your left ear towards your left shoulder as far as it is comfortable. Hold for 10–30 long slow breaths.

Cat stretch

This exercise will help to increase your spinal articulation. Repeat this exercise 3–6 times.

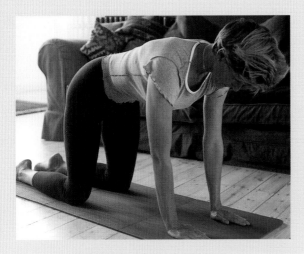

1 Start on your hands and knees, making sure that your hands are beneath your shoulders and your hips are above your knees. Make sure that your back is flat and your head and neck are in alignment with your back, parallel to the floor. Breathe in, sensing the breath coming in between your shoulder blades. Pull up your pelvic floor and pull in your stomach muscles.

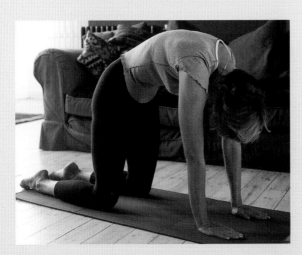

2 Breathing out, curl your tailbone underneath you, push into your hands and lift your breastbone, tucking your chin and then your head underneath. Hold this position and breathe in. Breathe out and lower yourself back into the starting position (step 1) by reversing the sequence, bringing your head back up to its position parallel with the floor, followed by your chin and finally your tailbone.

Get fit without the fuss!

There are lots of ways in which you can introduce more exercise into your lifestyle without making big changes, or having to join a gym.

- If your workplace is close to your home, you could get up a little earlier, leave your car at home and walk to work – you will be doing your bit for the environment that way as well!
- If you have a longer journey, get off the subway, bus or train two stops earlier. A brisk 20 minute walk each day is excellent for getting your heart pumping, and you will feel refreshed and energized when you start work.

If you don't want to join a formal exercise class, try visiting your local gym and using the exercise machines.

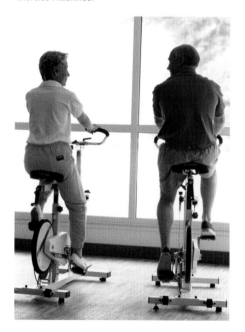

- Housework and gardening can both help you work up a sweat: push the vacuum that much harder, rake the lawn more energetically, and stretch up with that feather duster – it all makes a difference!
- Get into the habit of taking a lunchtime stroll. Just walking to the sandwich shop will boost your fitness levels, and help you avoid that post-lunchtime energy slump.
- If you work at home, theoretically it is easier to take a break, but in practice you need to discipline yourself to build in time for exercise. It helps to have a dog – dogs are always pleased to have an opportunity to go for walkies!
- Alternatively, you could exercise at home in front of an exercise video.
- If sexual intimacy is part of your life, then vigorous sex can be a great form of exercise, boosting your heart rate, increasing your lung capacity and giving your muscles a workout. However, sex may be the last thing on your mind until your menopausal symptoms are under control, and an understanding partner can make all the difference.
- If you are spending the day shopping, try walking between shopping areas, rather than jumping on the bus or taking the car – carrying bags is a good way to combine a walk with weight-bearing exercise.
- When you are shopping in a department store, take the stairs instead of the lift or escalator. Climbing stairs helps tone your leg muscles and raises your heart rate.
- Stretch, skip and jog for 5–10 minutes while you are watching the TV or listening to music.

COMMONSENSE PRECAUTIONS WHEN STARTING TO EXERCISE

- If you are over 50 and have health risk factors or have been extremely inactive, see your doctor before starting an exercise programme.
- Exercise must be regular. A weekend blitz – where your usual sedentary self suddenly leaps into six hours of tennis – is more dangerous than helpful.
- Stop if you feel short of breath, a muscle strain, joint pain, or numbness and tingling, especially in your chest and arms.
- Use the right shoes. Exercise has become shoe-specific, with walking shoes for walking, step shoes for step aerobics, and many kinds of running and aerobic dance shoes. You may be tempted to use the same pair for every activity, but an investment in proper shoes is essential – for the sake of your feet!
- Do not overlook the importance of sleep. If you are suffering menopausal night sweats, then your sleeping pattern will be totally out of kilter. It is important to try to catch up on sleep as and when you are able.
- If you need some instruction, get it. Books and videos can give you an idea of how to get started, but if you want to go past the basics, join a class.
- Drink a glass of water before and after exercising. Do not be tempted to rely on thirst as an indicator of how much water you need – if you are thirsty, you are already water-depleted.
- Sports such as golf, tennis, badminton, and cricket are fun and a great way to socialize, but because the nature of the sports requires you constantly to start and stop, they rarely keep your heart rate consistently high enough to qualify as aerobic exercise.

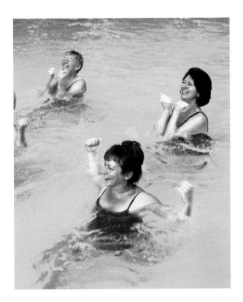

Find out about local exercise classes, you may be surprised at the amount of activities you can join in.

- If you want to build your stamina and maintain a healthy heart, then choose continuous-movement activities such as walking or swimming, or join an aerobic dance class.

SHOULD I EXERCISE WHEN I FEEL ILL?

If you have a headache, stuffy nose or you are sneezing, try exercising for 10 minutes, then evaluate how you feel. If you feel fine, continue. But if you have a chesty cough, stomach pain or muscle strain it's best to skip your exercise session for a day or two.

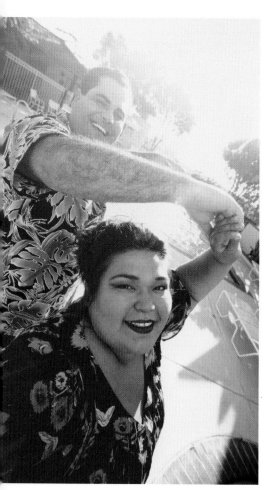

If you don't want to join your local gym,
why not try dancing lessons instead.

LET'S DANCE!

You may have holidayed abroad and returned with glowing memories of cultures in which dance is a vital part of life.

And what a choice we have worldwide! Where once social dancing was restricted to the traditional ballroom, nowadays clubs offering instruction in flamenco, lambada, line-dancing and breakaway swing (jiving plus a few solo moves) have sprung up all over the place, with salsa and Argentine tango particularly on the rise.

Dancing is an instinctive celebration of our physical state of life – we do it when we feel good, and we feel good when we do it. It puts us in touch with ourselves and with others – the touch of another person confirms we are real, we are alive.

An evening's dancing as is as good a form of exercise as a three-hour hike. Dancing:

- releases energy and emotion
- pumps blood up our legs, so it's good for our hearts
- keeps our brains tuned
- promotes supple posture and relaxation
- encourages self-confidence and a sense of achievement as we master a new skill
- gives us the opportunity to get up close and personal to a range of partners, in a setting where ability and enthusiasm transcend age, gender and class.

Whatever your choice of exercise – enjoy it! If the 'feel-good' factor is missing, then try something different.

---

6 6 *Nobody cares if you can't dance well. Just get up and dance. Great dancers are not great because of their technique, they are great because of their passion.*

MARTHA GRAHAM

US dancer and teacher (1895-1991) 9 9

Selected bibliography

CHAPTER 1

Ford, G. *Listening to Your Hormones*
Prima, 1996
Mason, A. *Health and Hormones* Penguin
Books, 1960
Melville, A. *Natural Hormone Health*
Thorsons, 1990
Sellman, S. *Hormone Heresy* Getwell
International, 2000
Teaff, N. and Wiley, K. *Perimenopause –
Preparing for the Change* Prima, 1999

CHAPTER 2

Clark, J. *Hysterectomy and the
Alternatives* Virago, 1993;
Vermilion, 2000
Clark, J. *HRT and the Natural Alternatives*
Hamlyn, 2003
Coney, S. *The Menopause Industry*
Spinifex Press Pty Ltd. Australia, 1991
Kenton, L. *Passage to Power* Vermilion,
1996
Ridley, M. *Genome – The Autobiography of
a Species in 23 Chapters* Fourth Estate,
1999

CHAPTER 3

Bradford, N. *The Hamlyn Encyclopaedia of
Complementary Health* Hamlyn, 2000
Glenville, M. *Natural Alternatives to HRT*
Kyle Cathie, 1997
Roland, P. *How to Meditate* Hamlyn, 2000
Simonton, O. C. *Getting Well Again*
Bantam Books, 1978
Whiteaker, S. *The Good Retreat Guide*
Rider, 2001

CHAPTER 4

Mervyn, L. *The Dictionary of Vitamins*
Thorsons, 1984
Norman, J. *Aromatic Herbs* Dorling
Kindersley, 1989
Savarin-Brillat, J. A. *The Physiology of
Taste* Penguin 1970 (First published
1825)

CHAPTER 5

Blount, T. and McKenzie, E. *PilateSystem*
Hamlyn, 2001

Index

Acknowledgements

Executive Editor: Jane McIntosh
Project Editor: Charlotte Wilson
Executive Art Editor: Leigh Jones
Designer: Tony Truscott
Picture Researcher: Luzia Strohmayer
Production Controller: Nosheen Shan

Illustrations: Philip Wilson, and Cactus Design and Illustration
Index: Indexing Specialists (UK) Ltd

Acestock Ltd 42, 48; **Alamy**/ Phoebe Dunn 14/ Imagestate 117/ Image Source 7; **Bubbles**/ Jennie Woodcock 49 right; **Getty Images**/ Samuel Ashfield 41/ Chris Cheadle 79/ Jim Cummins 36/ Candice Farmer 123/ Howard Grey 9, 13/ David Hanover 53/ Walter Hodges 109, 110/ Romilly Lockyer 111/ Stuart McClymont 124/ Laurence Monneret 18/ Antony Nagelmann 78/ Andreas Pollok 72/ Mark Scott 92/ Steve Smith 1, 47/ Terry Vine 15 /Mel Yates 88; **Octopus Publishing Group Limited** 3, 31, 71/ Colin Bowling 26, 62, 67 top, 67 bottom, 70/ Jean Cazals 106 left/ Colin Gotts 115/ Marcus Harpur 68 right/ Sandra Lane 102/ Sean Myers 68 left/ Peter Pugh-Cook 10, 25, 49 left, 63, 76, 81, 82, 86, 89, 114/ William Reavell 90, 93, 94 right, 97, 98 top, 103/ Gareth Sambidge 55, 83 top, 83 Centre, 83 bottom, 85/ Nikki Sianni 56, 74, 112, 113, 116/ Ian Wallace 4, 75, 87 top, 87 bottom, 94 left, 98 bottom, 104 left, 104 right, 105 left, 106 right/ Philip Webb 105 right/ Mark Winwood 2, 118, 119, 120, 121; **Science Photo Library**/ David Gifford 37/ Tim Malon & Paul Biddle 60 /Andrew McClenaghan 61/ Will & Deni McIntyre 34/ Professors P.M. Motta & J. Van Blerkom 17/ Perlstein, Jerrican 122/ Sinclair Stammers 32/ Tek Image 58/ Sheila Terry 64 bottom/ Th Foto-Werbung 64 Top/ Jim Varney 46/ Hattie Young 50; **Wellfoods Limited**/Tel: 01226 381 712/ www.bake-it.com 100.